The Best

You'll Ever Have

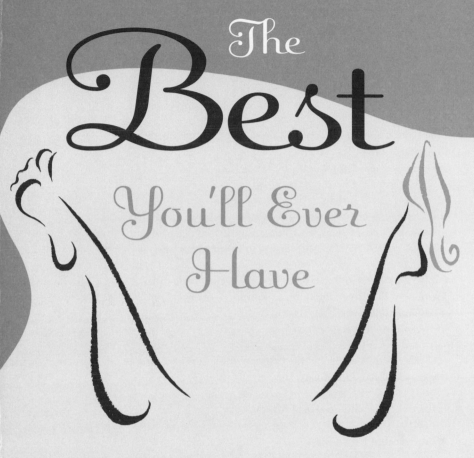

What Every Woman Should Know
about Getting and Giving

Knock-Your-Socks-Off Sex

SHANNON MULLEN

with Valerie Frankel

Illustrations by Sandy Haight

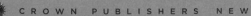

CROWN PUBLISHERS NEW YORK

Published by Crown Publishers, New York, New York.
Member of the Crown Publishing Group,
a division of Random House, Inc.
www.crownpublishing.com

CROWN is a trademark and the Crown colophon is a registered
trademark of Random House, Inc.

Printed in the United States of America

A Roundtable Press Book

For Roundtable Press, Inc.
Directors: Julie Merberg and Marsha Melnick
Design by Margo Mooney
Associate Editor: Sara Newberry

Library of Congress Cataloging-in-Publication Data is available
upon request.

ISBN-13: 978-1-4000-5482-4
ISBN-10: 1-4000-5482-6

10 9 8 7 6 5 4 3 2

First Edition

Contents

What's a Nice Girl Like Me Doing in the Sex Toy Business?

While checking out this book at the bookstore, you probably glanced at my photo on the back. As you see, I am a normal-looking woman: Midwesternish, midthirties, auburn hair, straight teeth. Not homely, but not a knockout either (although I do my best). I don't have deep cleavage, big teased blonde hair, a leather dress, or latex underpants. Nor do I look like a shrink with fifty years of couples counseling under my belt. I probably look like someone you know. I may even look like you. I may *be* like you— an interesting, curious, happy person, if somewhat ordinary. Until a few years ago, I worked at an advertising agency, went to dinner with friends, dated whenever I got the chance, and looked forward to the week- ends and my next vaca- tion. A typical American woman.

I'm not quite so typical anymore. Most American women don't sell sex toys for a living. But more are joining me every day because lots of women buy them— or should. I've learned that much since the creation of Safina, the company I founded to provide sex information and products for women. I'm now an official, if unorthodox, "sexpert." Unlike the majority of sexperts, I have never appeared in a porn movie. I don't do inner sex goddess classes with hand mirrors and chanting. I haven't hosted couples retreats in the mountains where I advise lovers to gaze into each other's

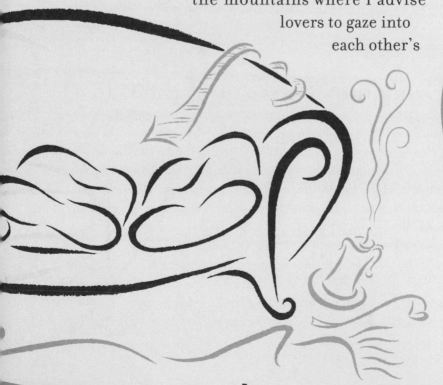

eyes and breathe in sync. You will never hear me spouting new age psychobabble about sexuality. My approach is the result of my personal, I dare say, typical sexual experience as a civilian—not a professional—sexual being, and a lot of research.

That said, I have also presided over hundreds of Safina Salons (more on Salons later), I've spoken with and lectured to thousands of women nationwide about sex, and I've conducted seminars and classes through the Learning Annex and other organizations on how women can improve their sexual pleasure. I've made gathering sexual information job one and have interviewed dozens of groundbreaking doctors and researchers in the United States and beyond. I've studied the history of sex from the ancient Greeks to modern presidents. For the last few years, my life has been all sex research, all the time. My life has made a 180-degree turn since my days as an advertising executive. It all began—the idea to start the company, and to devote myself to sexual education—with a question. A question that is common to most women but that often goes unasked. If Safina does nothing more (although it does—much, much more), I hope we adequately address the query, "Am I normal?"

Dragging Sex Out of the Closet

I was living in Brussels for an advertising job when the President Clinton/ Monica Lewinsky sex scandal broke. The Europeans were bewildered by our government's reaction to the scandal. I was constantly asked to explain why our government cared about our president's sex life when the women he saw were clearly over 18 and consenting. When I returned to New York, I noticed a concrete shift in our culture. Sex was a topic of open discussion on TV and in restaurants. Of course, people talked about sex before. But I'd never heard newscasters saying "oral sex" previously or Barbara Walters asking Ms. Lewinsky if the president made her "as a woman, happy and content." It was my turn to be shocked. Meanwhile, *Sex and the City* was not just beloved in New York as it had been when I left, but it had become wildly popular all over the country. The ribald honesty of the characters made Madonna's formerly shocking behavior seem quaint in comparison. Victoria's Secret had boomed in my absence too and was now having runway shows broadcast on network TV with their "Very Sexy" collection, which was more Frederick's of Hollywood than their formerly Victorian style. Staid magazines like *Redbook*, once full of recipes and mommy tips, now blazed tantalizing cover lines that were just as raunchy as *Cosmopolitan*.

You turn your back on a country for two years and look what happens! While I was gone, sex had moved to the forefront of the American culture agenda. And yet, when I met my girlfriends for drinks and the subject turned to their own sex lives, all I heard were the same vague statements they'd always made like, "My new boyfriend is awesome in bed." No one spoke as explicitly, it seemed, as Ms. Lewinsky, and she did so only under subpoena. The new national openness was great in the abstract, but on a woman-to-woman level, sexuality remained a sealed state secret.

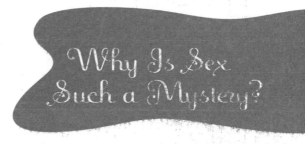

Why Is Sex Such a Mystery?

Eating is essential for survival, like breathing, drinking, and sex. What could be more essential for our species' survival than sex? We know a lot about how to eat, breathe, and drink. And although everyone can recite reproductive mechanics, you'd be surprised by the huge educational gaps in basic sexual anatomy and the physiology of pleasure. Don't believe me? Tell me then, how long is the clitoris (answer on page 35)? What's the difference between the vulva and vagina (see page 23)? Where and what is the prostate (see pages 89–93)? The perineum (page 96)? What are the four stages of arousal (pages 73–77)? I could go on (in fact, I do—for the rest of this book). We are all interested in sex, fascinated by it, obsessed with it. So why don't we know everything there is to know about our bodies and what they can do? What's standing in the way?

I'm convinced that the gap is due to how information is presented— as either too medical sounding and therefore impersonal or too explicit and therefore embarrassing. Sleazy sex book covers can be downright mortifying. I've long felt that buying one would reflect negatively on me (although who would care anyway? Strangers and cashiers?). Sex toy packaging and the dark, shady stores where you buy the stuff are even more off-putting. Even the outsides of those stores are sleazy. Why aren't sex toys presented like cosmetics or lacy underwear instead of deviant gizmos for hookers? Sex equals sleaze in our consumer culture (and in our creative culture). No wonder people hesitate before seeking information and buying products or admitting the naked truth to their friends.

Hesitancy about sex dovetails into hesitancy about talking about sex with a partner. If I had a nickel for every time a woman told me, "If I tell him what I want him to do to me in bed, he'll think I'm 'slutty' or 'greedy' or 'demanding,'" well, I'd be drowning in nickels. It's amazing that women can tell a hairstylist or a waiter in precise detail how to trim their bangs or cook their food, but women can't bring themselves to say "not there, *there*" to the most important person in their lives.

I believe that open, honest, straightforward talk should be the norm in all relationships. This must include sex talk. Otherwise, you carry on, not enjoying sex as much as you could. Resentment and/or boredom grow. The result: isolation within a relationship. It seems contradictory to have fear and silence in a love union. It's not healthy, but as I've learned, it is typical.

When I was in my early twenties, I had a boyfriend who was enthusiastic in bed, but he had the attention span of a flea. He'd leap from one thing to the next too quickly. I'd just be getting into his hand motions when he'd suddenly change pace or completely stop to start something else. It was unsatisfying for me, but he seemed to be having a great time. "I should be enjoying this," I kept thinking. He was doing his best, after all. In frustration, I tried to keep him on track by saying, "That feels fantastic" and "That's perfect." But he didn't take the hint. It must be me, I decided. I take too long to get into a groove. It's my fault. I vowed to just get used to it. I didn't get the chance though. He dumped me for an ex-girlfriend. I was stunned. Our sex life didn't come up in the "it's not you, it's me" exit interview, but I wondered if he knew it wasn't good for me. His no-longer-ex must have been happy with his style. The fault rested in my lap. Again, something was wrong with me.

The end of a relationship always raises questions. You can see why I was busy asking myself, "Am I normal?" at the conclusion of this one. I decided that the matter was too important to wonder about. If I was ever going to have the kind of open, honest relationship I wanted I knew I'd have to figure out what normal was and how to better communicate. So I set about learning everything I could about relationships and sex. I talked openly with a few close friends about these issues, and I found out that they had the same problems and concerns. When I saw that our culture was shifting to a more open discussion about sex, I knew that I could help make that discussion happen. I was sure there was a lot of information out there that needed to be made more accessible. I read every book I could find about sex and relationships (still do). I attended workshops and interviewed gynecologists and urologists. I read medical journals and talked to the doctors who authored the studies. I interviewed every type of sex worker. I'm social by nature. I can talk to anyone, about anything. I've found that no topic interests people as much as sex. Once people see you as a nonjudgmental, interested stranger, they'll tell you anything—far more than they'll tell friends— and it was all very fascinating and informative.

Meanwhile, all of this research cut severely into my day job at the advertising agency. So I quit. I took a deep breath and called my mother and told her what I'd done. "Great," she said. "What are you going to do?" Suddenly I realized that she thought I'd landed a bigger, better advertising job at another agency. I didn't know what to say.

I'd never talked to her about sex since we'd had "the talk" when I was a kid. Nervous as hell, I blurted out, "I'm going to start a business. For women. A sex information and sex toy business. Not sleazy. Like something you've never seen. In the same format as Mary Kay or Tupperware but high-end. Sophisticated and affordable. Chic and smart. Useful information and pretty products. Nice packaging." Mom said nothing. I'd stunned her silent. "Are you still there?" I asked terrified that she'd hung up.

"I'm here," she said. "I'm just thinking about it. You know, I think it could work." She actually believed that my company could fill a need in the marketplace. I can't tell you how important her support has been to me.

Most of my female friends and coworkers cheered me on too. But my straight male friends and associates (and, it followed, many of the bankers and investors I sought out for financing) thought I'd lost my mind. They didn't see what need my business would fulfill, and they didn't believe women would want to host Safina Salons in their living rooms. And they definitely didn't think I'd sell anything or be able to find salespeople. I heard the same "It'll never fly" dozens of times from men. Each time, I have to admit, it hurt.

But they were wrong. I eventually found an important supporter who believed in my idea—my dear friend John. John had experience starting up small businesses. His guidance and confidence kept me going (John, this is my official "thank you a million times, I couldn't have done it without you"). With his business-end support, I devoted myself completely to my sexual education. And that quickly evolved into the pursuit of educating others.

A Company Is Born

After my book research, I had to go into the field to buy and sample sex toys. To inspire me, I bought a big blue dildo and kept it on my desk. I stared at it when I was on the phone and as I collected the product sources and catalogs. It startled me when I entered and left the room at first. It was so big, so blue, so penis-like. When the doorbell rang, I'd hurl it into the closet. After a few days though, I got used to it. My cleaning lady, however, wasn't prepared for the shock.

"Oh my god!" she screamed when she came in and saw it for the first time.

"What?" I asked. Immediately, I saw where her bugged-out eyes were staring. I was mortified. My newfound comfort level was shattered. "Oh, Lisa, don't worry about that," I said. "It's for my new job. I work at home now."

She looked at me with rank horror.

I realized what I'd just said.

I said, "Wait a minute. You don't think I'm working *with* that, at home?" I shook my head. "No, it's not like that."

She tilted her head now. Very confused. I picked up the dildo and said, "It's just plastic. I'm going to sell these to women who need them."

Lisa had heard more than enough. She said, "I don't want to know. I'll just dust. You get out of here and I'll just dust."

A few weeks later, my mantle was crammed with sex toys from all over the world. I'd been buying each and every sex appliance I could find and was gathering quite a collection (eventually honed way down for Safina's catalogue). I came home one afternoon just as Lisa was leaving "Okay, I'm ready to listen now. What is this new job?" she asked.

I sat her down and explained things. Shocked as she'd been when she first saw Big Blue, it couldn't have equaled my surprise when Lisa asked if I could recommend a product for her. As soon as she asked, I knew I was in the right business.

Talk to Me

I developed Safina Sex-Ed Salons for women so that I could teach women about anatomy and physiology and introduce them to toys in a comfortable, nurturing environment (that is, someone's living room and not a gross, dark wrong-side-of-the-tracks porn store). What ultimately transpired: I learned just as much from the women I thought I was educating as they learned from me. I was starting to get a firm answer to the question that started it all, sorting out "normal" as I went along.

The women-only Salons are parties in people's living rooms. Cheese and wine are served, and the Safina Specialist leads a discussion about sex. Like at Tupperware parties, the Safina rep brings samples of various sex toys to show women what they are and what they can do. I've heard people refer to our Salons as "fuckerware parties," which doesn't capture the tone of them at all, and sounds crass to boot. There is a sales component, but our Salons are about much more than hawking product.

Safina Salons combine sex information with storytelling. We introduce a subject, say, the G-spot, and a roomful of women start swapping the tales of their adventures. The Salons are always funny, surprising, exciting, and liberating. The more I did, the more I heard common themes in women's stories. Once they are comfortable, the guests told stories of confusion and fumbling, of sudden discoveries and intimate confessions. Friends who have known the confessors for years would shout, "I didn't know that!" and "You never told me that before" and then launch into stories of their own. The silence around sex was broken. Smiles and laughs would burst forth. Talking about anatomy, technique, and how to tell your guy what you want isn't just a fun way to pass an evening. It's useful. It sweeps away the shame, and everyone leaves a Salon feeling energized, connected, and exhilarated (and often ready for action).

Over time, I got the Web site off the ground (www.safina.com), acquired a warehouse, and set up professional shipping. I started to build a national sales force of Safina Specialists who do Safina Salons in their areas. We continue to grow even in states where you'd think people didn't even have sex, much less talk about it.

The Oldest Thing in the World Is Still New

Better sit-ups are always being invented. It's hard to believe that with all our technology and medical advances, we haven't mastered our understanding of stomach muscles. Just goes to show you: we're continuously improving and upgrading. The human body is complicated. The established "best" ways to feed it and develop it change all the time. Think of nutrition: ten years ago, it was low fat. Nuts were evil and bacon would kill you. Two years ago, it was low carb, with nuts and bacon on top of the To Eat list. Now, the movement is heading back toward low fat. You can see shifts in everything, every style and invention. Ten years ago, luggage didn't have wheels without tipping over. Wrinkles didn't have Botox. The world of invention and education never stops spinning. If there's always going to be a better kitchen gadget, there will always be new ideas about sex.

I am convinced, however, that the most progress we can make in discovering more about sex is by talking to each other. If we shared our stories with our friends on a regular basis, we'd reduce the amount of stumbling around and stressful trial and error that we all go through. Our collective knowledge and confidence would rise along with our happiness. Back to the idea of "normal": if you knew for sure that each of your friends shared your sexual quirks or desires, you wouldn't feel unsettled about them, would you? It's human nature to fear being different, while at the same time, Americans prize individuality. It's complicated. But much less so if we air out our concerns. *Making sex a normal, everyday topic erases fear and doubt.* Knowing that you are normal, as it turns out, has an enormous effect on how you see yourself, how you enjoy sex, and how close you feel to your partner.

You Decide What's Normal

In intimate relationships, women are the gatekeepers of physical intimacy. If you think about it, this makes perfect sense since we are the ones whose bodies can change as a result of that intimacy. But this simple fact extends to how relationships work overall. Women are often the moral compasses of relationships. We tend to be the leaders in opinions on what is and isn't acceptable or nice. Even when I was in school I could see this. The kids who really determined girls' reputations weren't the boys, but the other girls.

In order to change how sexuality is viewed in society, we must start with how women see things. Where sex is concerned, it is both our traditional role and our biological imperative to be cautious. Caution often determines what we will and won't let happen with our partners, even when it comes to conversation and exploration.

This book is a first step toward normalizing any sexual conversation and exploration. Men need a lot of education, and they need to change their thinking as well, and they're next. But because women take a leadership role in intimacy, I want to address women first. (If you are a lesbian, I hope you'll overlook the heterosexual bias in how this book is written. I don't mean to offend.)

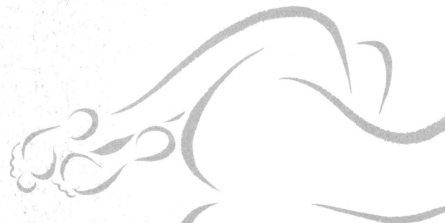

> ## "If sex is such a natural phenomenon, how come there are so many books on how to do it?" —Bette Midler

"Sex comes naturally" doesn't ring true. "Nature" is an idealized myth buried under many layers of our culture, including our own experiences, media, relationships, education, and so on. Everything must be learned, from math to reading to blow-drying our hair—and sex is no different. As I've already mentioned, the huge gaps in our sexual education (fear, shame, silence, etc.) shorten the learning curve. Harry Truman said, "There is nothing new in the world except the history you do not know." So it seems to me that you might as well build on other people's sexual learning curves, which might be steeper than yours.

I'd say my curve is pretty damn steep. I'm going to give you all I've got. I'll be delicate yet candid and hopefully not off-putting, although that can be hard to accomplish. Talking about sex can be shocking or embarrassing. Even someone with an open mind will blush when exposed to words that usually go unmentioned. But momentary embarrassment seems like a very small price to pay in exchange for learning how to expand our pleasure horizons and giving our partners new experiences that will get better and better as we boldly go where few women have gone before.

I trust that you'll be able to relate to my experiences as well as identify with the women's stories I've collected along the way. I also hope that you'll feel confident enough to share your own thoughts and ideas with me via e-mail at comments@safina.com or at a Safina Salon. This book—part autobiography, part history, with real stories and voices throughout—is as much a conversation as it is a concrete, practical sex guide (including all the signposts and directions needed to take you where you want to go). Ideally, my conversational style will launch many frank discussions with your friends. Whether these talks start with the question, "Am I normal?" or not, the conclusions will be the same. This book will prove that you are not alone and that you are normal.

The C Word

Show of hands. Who remembers hearing the word "clitoris" in fifth grade sex-ed class? Anyone? I sure didn't. I first heard this particular C word in college, circa 1990 (I'd heard the other C word way before then and hadn't liked the sound of it one bit). I didn't get a long hard look at a clitoris until my late 20s, and that was the one I had on me. Since I hadn't seen any others, I was surprised by what I saw in the hand mirror. It was small and red and oddly shaped, if I was even looking at the right part. I worried I might be deformed. The whole area looked misshapen. *Now* I know that most women have this same fear and that none of us are deformed. But my sexual education took decades, starting with my fifth grade health class.

Chapter 2

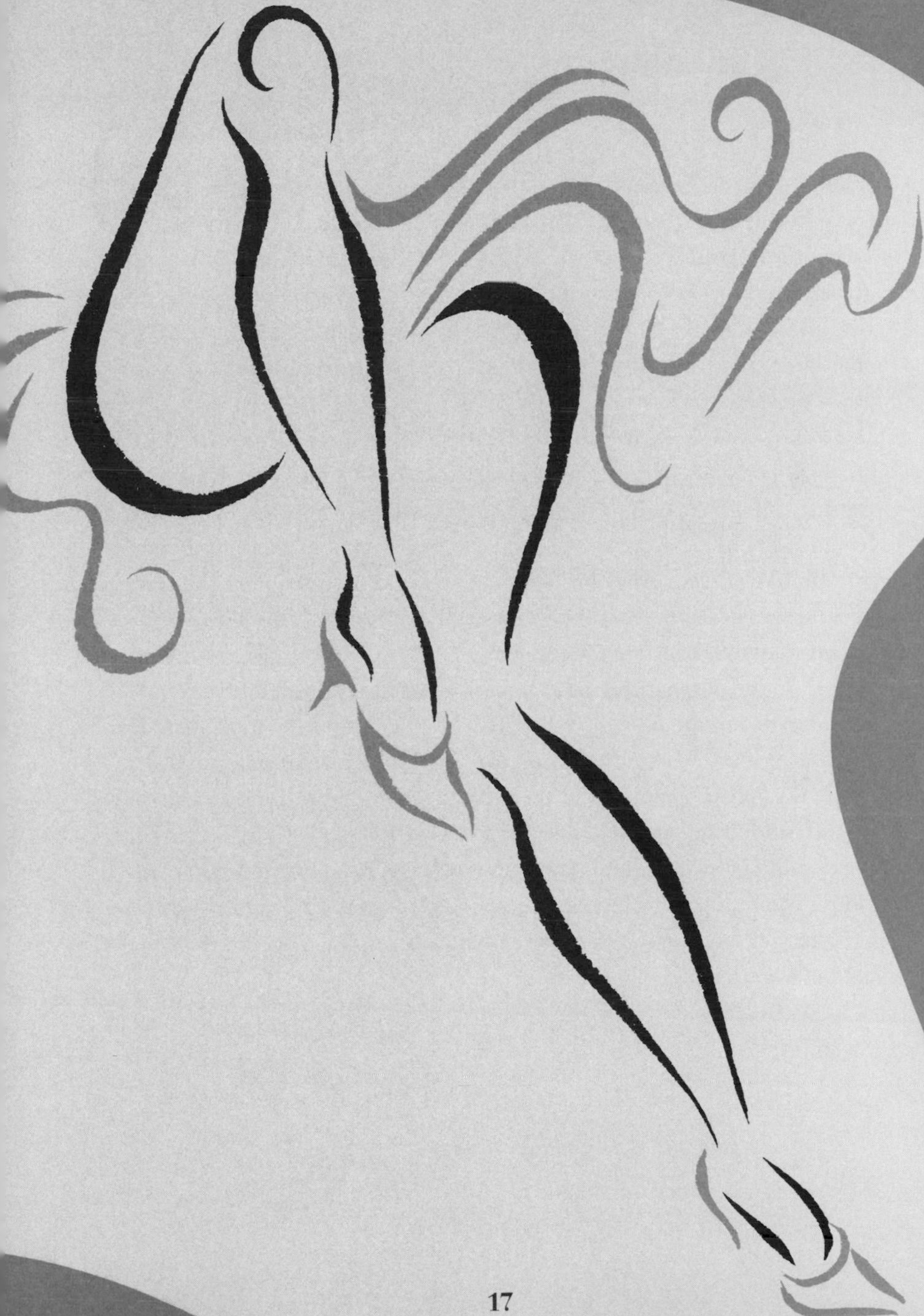

Are You There God?
It's Me, Shannon

When I was 10, the only books that really resonated with me and my friends were written by Judy Blume. Her novels were the most sympathetic and informative books I'd encountered, and I'm still grateful to her for making me feel normal in my preteen confusion. I could have easily placed myself into any of her plots, but the one character that hit home the hardest with me—and millions of other girls—was Margaret.

I read *Are You There God? It's Me, Margaret* a dozen times in fifth grade. My copy was dog-eared and tattered, but I kept going back to it, paging through certain parts on a nearly daily basis. Margaret and her friends were all getting their periods and kissing boys. I was fascinated.

On the last morning of school that year, just hours before the start of summer vacation, the school nurse, Mrs. Blanche, came into my homeroom and made an announcement. All the girls were to go down the hall to the other fifth grade classroom; all the boys should stay put and were to be joined by the other fifth grade boys for health class today.

We all knew what was coming. We'd gotten to the human sexuality chapter in our textbook. We'd seen the curious illustrations and already learned about the sperm and the egg the week before. As my friends and I walked down the hall to join the other girls, we were nervous and giddy. The mysteries of the universe were about to be cracked open. Secrets would be revealed. Darkness and confusion would turn to the light of knowledge. Or so we thought.

What Every Girl Should Know

As we found seats, Mrs. Blanche started a filmstrip called "What Every Girl Should Know." When the filmstrip got to the female anatomy—a chart of the ovaries, fallopian tubes, and uterus (the same illustration that was in the textbooks)—Mrs. Blanche paused the film and pointed out the parts, talked about the movement of the eggs once a month, and explained menstruation in a very straightforward and reassuring way. Then she handed out little kits that we were to take home. She patiently explained the contents of the kit. There was a pad for when we got our periods—in a pink plastic pouch, along with a pink booklet, also called "What Every Girl Should Know." I flipped through it. More ovaries. Another uterus.

And then the class was over. I was happy to get the little kit to take home, but the pads scared me. They were bulky, big as a brick, and surely visible through jeans, despite what Mrs. Blanche said. Unlike Margaret, I wasn't quite as eager to begin life as a woman. Getting my period sounded messy, uncomfortable, and terrifyingly grown-up. And what if I got mine before the other girls? I became worried that it would set me apart or mark me for ridicule.

But the biggest disappointment about the class was that Mrs. Blanche failed to explain anything I was really interested in. Ovaries and blood had nothing to do with love and excitement. I wanted to understand the feeling I had when I thought about kissing a boy. What was going on in movies between men and women? Is this all there was?

I went home and reread "What Every Girl Should Know" while locked in the upstairs bathroom. I wondered how badly cramps would hurt and how much blood there would be. I thought about the potential mortification of running in gym class with that huge pad in my underwear or leaking all over the basketball court. Perhaps it would be best, I thought, if the secrets and mysteries of sex were left undiscovered.

Fear, confusion, dread. Not an auspicious way to begin a sex life. Mrs. Blanche hadn't fallen down on her duty. It goes without saying that the transactions between sperm and egg taught me about reproduction.

But her class didn't prepare me at all for SEX. Besides my beloved Judy Blume books (which, aside from *Forever*—remember Ralph the penis?—hardly went beyond second base), my adolescent knowledge of sex came from the beauty parlor's stack of *Glamour* and *Cosmopolitan* magazines that my mother never bought. But the articles inside were frustratingly cryptic and raised more questions than answers. To this day, twenty years later, women's magazines continue to serve up the requisite "How to Drive Your Man Wild" and "Am I normal?" stories each month. Most of us, even as adults it seems, are still wondering what sex is about, having a hardtime finding answers, and wondering if we're deformed.

Who Says Ignorance Is Bliss?

After talking to hundreds of women at Safina Salons, I realize now that I was lucky to get any sex-ed at all. I frequently meet women in their late 20s who thought they had cancer or were dying when their period started because no one told them what to expect. Tanya, a 30-year-old mother of two, told me her horror story:

I was 12, sitting in class, and felt an odd dripping sensation in my underwear. I looked down and saw a huge red blotch on my white shorts. I felt complete panic but managed to calmly get up and leave the room without asking permission. I was too scared to speak! I went straight to lost and found, found a pair of pants that fit, and went to the bathroom. When I undressed and saw the blood, I assumed I was dying. I didn't know what to do or who could help me. I balled up the shorts, put them between my legs, pulled the pants on over them, and finished the day at school, knowing I had one week to live. When I got home, my grandmother explained it all. But that'll go down as one of the most terrifying afternoons of my life.

This story blows me away every time I'm reminded of it. What's even more mind-blowing: Tanya isn't unique in her first period experience. I've heard variations on this story again and again. Hard to believe in the twenty-first century, isn't it?

Call It the American Paradox

You've heard of the French paradox, how they can eat pounds of cheese in a single sitting and guzzle rich cream sauces by the bucketfull, yet they remain skinny nonetheless? Well, we have a paradox in the United States too. Our countrymen and countrywomen are obsessed with sex, yet the introduction to our sex lives is mired in embarrassment and confusion. Even though we have the most sex of any industrialized nation (even more than the thin, well-fed, sexy French), we are still misinformed about it. We are saturated by images of naked women, and yet few American females have even looked at their own private parts.

Show of hands. Who has held a hand mirror under their naked butt to see what's going on down there? Anyone? I often wondered what I looked like "down there," years before I actually took a peek. Once when I was around 8, I started to peel off my leotard after dance class with the idea of trying to see myself in the full-length mirror hanging on the back of my bedroom door. I didn't even get it off both shoulders when my sister walked in, guessed in an instant what I was trying to do, looked at me with sheer disgust, and left. I was embarrassed and ashamed. I quickly dressed and didn't dare try to glance between my legs for fifteen more years.

My sister's attitude definitely discouraged my healthy curiosity about that region of my body. But she merely contributed to the message I'd been picking up over the years: "Don't look, don't ask, don't touch." I suppose the silence around sex started in the earliest stages of life. I would ask, "Why is the sky blue?" and get a thoughtful response. But if I asked, "Where does pee come from?" or "What's a penis," I met with some very uptight reactions or was told to stop asking. Good girls were supposed to wipe from front to back and that was it. There wasn't even a name for what we were wiping.

In hosting Safina Salons, I've met only one woman, Jessica, who had a long, informative conversation with her parents when she was 10 on the subjects of anatomy and how the body and mind react during sex. She is the only one in thousands of women. When I demanded to know what tampons were for (I was probably 9), my own mother refused to answer me until we'd left the supermarket and were alone on the living room couch. She said, "When you get older, women bleed, right here." She was patting her inner thigh, on the seam of her jeans, as she talked. "It doesn't hurt. The tampon is for absorbing the flow." From that day forward, or until Judy Blume came into my life, I believed a gash would spontaneously appear on every woman's right inner thigh and bleed until it healed itself. Like a cut from a scissors, but not from scissors. What was I supposed to think?

With such silence and confusion about sex in our childhoods, it's a wonder we can ever take control and gain confidence in the erotic realm as adults. If sexual functioning were treated as practically and perfunctorily as, say, eating or sleeping, we'd all be far better off. When I think about the time and energy that was wasted unlearning what I'd been told, and then learning the truth about my own anatomy and my sexual response, I often get angry. Why should any of us suffer in confusion and silence about sex when it's as basic and necessary to our health and happiness as good sleep and nutrition? That said, onward, to the center of female power: the clitoris, at last.

Open Wide

Okay, so when you were a kid, everything between your legs was untouchable, unspeakable, invisible, and unknowable. By hook or by crook, you get to know yourself anyway, and hopefully you still are. It should be an ongoing process. You are constantly changing. You probably study your hair, face, pores, belly, and butt in the mirror every day, scrupulously looking for change (fatter, slimmer, fine lines, gray strands). The vulva gets short shrift. If you look at it at all, it's probably not half as often as you twist around uncomfortably to see how your butt is doing.

Well, I'm proposing that you treat your nether regions with as much interest and respect as you pay to your skin or your hair—which, incidentally, gives you pleasure only when it's not too humid. The clitoris will give you pleasure in the rain, snow, sleet, hail, at any time of day or night. The first step to having such a dependable relationship is getting up close and personal.

The Vulva

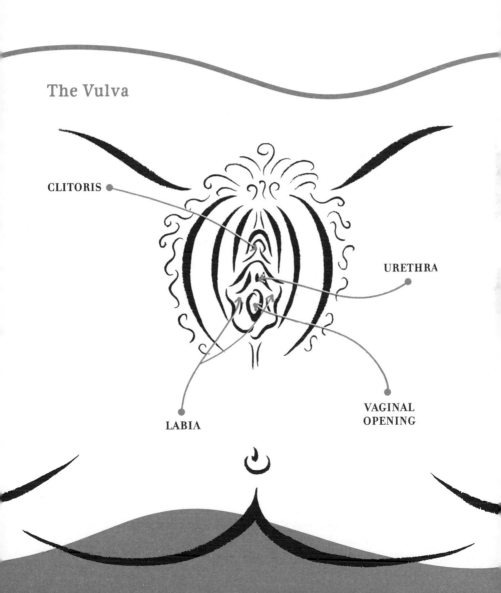

CLITORIS

URETHRA

LABIA

VAGINAL
OPENING

A Place for Everything, and Everything in Its Place

My daughter is 8 years old. We have her in a very progressive school where she's encouraged to ask questions about anything, which the teachers answer factually. She came home the other day from school and asked me if I knew that pee comes from one hole but that there are two others holes in girls. I wasn't sure she was right about there being three orifices, so I said, "Is that so?" Then I called my friend, who's 42 like me, and she told me that my daughter is right. I always thought we peed from the same place as the vagina. I'm mortified. How can I be this old, have two kids, and not know anything about my own body?"

—Jan, 42

Jan told me this story two years ago, at one of my first Salons. I was shocked—but not nearly as shocked as Jan was to learn the truth, and the degree of her own ignorance. Again, not to beat this point to death, but *she is not alone in being misinformed.* In fact, all the misinformation I came across in Salons led me to triple-check my own information. If I wanted to teach women about this stuff, I wanted to be sure I knew as much as I could inside and out, as it were. I plowed into research like a maniac.

This is what I learned: regarding the clitoris, some of the most famous modern medical literature might as well have been written in the Stone Age. This is a slight exaggeration, but only slight. The ancient Greeks understood the clitoris and its importance for female pleasure. They considered it a junior (and therefore inferior) equivalent to the penis. In the intervening thousands of years, knowledge of the clitoris and female pleasure shifted as attitudes toward women experiencing pleasure shifted. In the early 1900s, medical experts agreed with Freud that women should get their pleasure from intercourse—not their clitoris (fundamentally this meant that the in-out motion men so enjoyed equaled sex and women should like it the same way men did).

At the same time, few people thought it dignified if a woman really enjoyed sex. Men were considered animalistic and women were supposed to be above that. So a lot of cultural beliefs got in the way of knowing what good sex is from a woman's standpoint.

The anatomy of the clitoris wasn't even considered. The fact that it's more like a penis than not and wants the same amount of attention couldn't be accepted until our culture changed. At the turn of the century, people thought women ought to wear corsets and long dresses to play tennis and didn't see a connection between the corsets and women fainting—instead, they chalked it up to women being "the weaker sex." Clearly a lot had to change to face the fact that women like sex and can be just as "animalistic" about it if their pleasure is being attended to and they are allowed to be themselves.

Compounding the cultural blinders, the physiology of the clitoris wasn't high on the top of researchers' priority list at a time when doctors were dealing with issues like the search for a cure for scarlet fever (penicillin was only discovered in 1929) and a lot of other illnesses that we rarely get now. Julie Egan, curator of the Human Mind and Body Program in Australia, explains that the early diagrams of women's anatomy done during the Renaissance were based on only three females—a six-year-old child who'd been exhumed and two criminals who were executed. These drawings were the standard for a very long time.

By the early twentieth century, science was booming and progressing by leaps and bounds but the morality of the Victorian times deemed the clitoris unsuitable for research. It isn't necessary for reproduction; it doesn't get sick. The only problem seemed to be keeping little girls from touching it (masturbation was also considered an illness). Oddly, the cure for the main female illness in adult women was to stimulate the clitoris. This condition, called "hysteria," was considered the main cause of female troubles for the first half of the twentieth century. Doctors believed that the womb often became unmoored and wandered around a woman's body, causing her to be very emotional. To calm the symptoms, the clitoris was often treated manually or with vibratory devices in the doctor's office. (Yes, doctors would actually masturbate these women's symptoms away, but if women touched themselves, they were sick). The fact that this doctor-applied clitoral stimulation calmed down lots of "hysterical" women and that orgasms made these "sick" women feel better didn't add up to a diagnosis of sexual frustration to doctors back then. But then perception is reality. Facts don't stand a chance against deep-seated beliefs.

As recently as the 1960s and 1970s, after the "wandering womb" beliefs were refuted, doctors were still diagnosing American women with "frigidity" if they didn't have orgasms during standard missionary position sex. Their husbands, backed up by science, declared these, the majority of women (80 percent of them), defective. Women's feelings of inadequacy with their husbands were compounded when they went to the doctor only to be told they were indeed sick and were often put on drugs. Since muscle relaxants aren't magic orgasm-producing pills, women's problems were perpetual. Years of masturbation prohibition (pleasuring oneself was still thought to cause insanity and severed hands) made the sexually frustrated women feel much worse.

Luckily those days are over. It's incredible to think that all this misinformation was so recent. This dark history is part of why so few of us talk about sex today and why the clitoris remains shrouded in mystery.

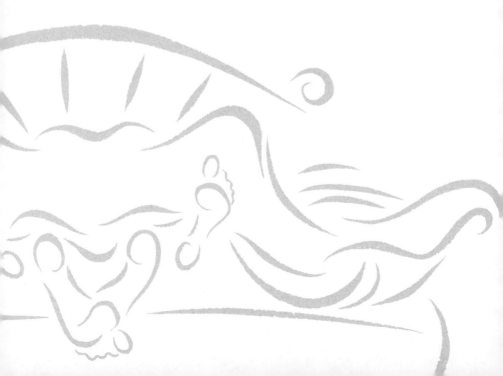

Can We Talk?

THE STORIES TOLD IN SAFINA SALONS MAKE WOMEN LAUGH, NOD IN RECOGNITION, OR SPONTANEOUSLY SHOUT OUT, "OH, NO!" IN EMPATHY OR SURPRISE. YOU MAY HAVE SIMILAR STORIES OF YOUR OWN. CHANCES ARE YOU HAVEN'T TOLD A SOUL. HERE ARE A FEW OF OTHER WOMEN'S STORIES OF THEIR BIG SECRETS VIS-À-VIS THE CLITORIS.

A LITTLE TRIM

I was afraid of waxing my bikini area, so I thought I'd just do a little trim and eliminate some of the excess. I got out my manicure scissors, which are very sharp. I sat on the edge of the bed and started snipping away. I thought my pubic hair did look better shorter. And then my hand slipped. I felt a sharp, intense, blinding-white sudden pain. I pressed down on the whole area in a panic, but when I took a quick look, I saw blood. I couldn't look after that. I started to cry. I was too scared to examine the extent of the damage. I was in serious pain. Terrified, I couldn't move.

My boyfriend heard me and came rushing in. I felt so stupid. There I was, sitting on the side of the bed with my robe open, hands pressing down, looking up at him. He knelt down and held my shoulders and asked so sweetly, "What's wrong? What's going on?" I couldn't speak I was crying so hard.

"I ... cut ... my ... clitoris," I gasped.

He said, "Let me see." I didn't want to let go. He got a wet towel and wiped me off and took a good look and then his tone changed completely, "You didn't cut your clitoris," he said. "You just nicked the hood a tiny bit. Take a look."

"What hood?" I asked. He gave me a hand mirror and showed me the clitoral hood and the clitoris underneath and the urethra and the vagina. I didn't even know there was a hood—and mine is huge. It's like a folded flap of skin. If you pull it back, and he did, you can see the clitoris. I'd taken a mirror and looked maybe once or twice before that, but I never thought to pull back the skin. I thought the flap *was* the clitoris. So here's my boyfriend, the same age as me, who'd been with me for four or five years since the middle of college, explaining my body parts to me. I felt so foolish and embarrassed. At the same time, I was so glad I hadn't cut my clitoris. I'd thought I'd never be able to fix it, that I'd never be able to enjoy sex again. So one minute I was thinking I'm doomed, and the next, my boyfriend is taking me on a tour of my vulva.

I demanded to know how he knew so much. He said, "I took an interest. I've read books. I can't believe you never wanted to know about yourself."

I couldn't believe it either. I've since taken a real interest, and that's why I became a Safina Specialist. I knew that if I could be so clueless there had to be others in the same state.   — Shameka, 29

MAGIC FINGERS

You know what amazes me about my clitoris? The time I wasted on men who didn't know what to do with it. It took me 32 years to find a man who knew how to touch it. I figured out a long time ago when I was a little girl that if I barely touched it, it felt amazing. I knew to start up higher, near my bone, not directly on the clitoris. I knew that if someone else did it, it would feel even better. But no one ever took enough time. I'd say, "Barely touch me," and the guy would zero in and press down and then massage like I had a muscle kink that needed kneading.

I'd try not to shriek at them, but it was awful. It was painful. I know I should've shown them what to do. I should've talked to them about it before we got in bed. But I always hoped the next guy would know what to do and that he'd listen to me when I told him to barely touch me.

I met Mike when I was 32. I really liked him. On our third date (the sex date), I was nervous about what would happen. When we got in bed, Mike's fingers were feather light. He started at my stomach and he made circles and wavy lines almost in the air above me. Even when he got close to the clitoris, he didn't change his approach. The light touches gave me shivers. I couldn't believe a sensation could be so overwhelmingly good. Pure happiness shot through me. It was the best sex of my life. It was a deal-sealer. A *deal-sealer!* We got married two and a half years later.   —Laura, 35

CLOSE ENCOUNTERS OF THE FIRST KIND

The first time a boy touched my clitoris was when I was about 9 or 10 years old. He was a kid my age. His family was staying in the hotel my family owns. I don't know how exactly I came to be lying down with him massaging me. I'm sure we were playing doctor (had to be that), but I don't remember any details—except how his hand felt on top of my shorts. Fantastic. I didn't know he was touching my clitoris and I don't even know if he knew. I was just astonished that anything could feel so good. I didn't move or speak in case he'd stop.

I thought about that afternoon a lot afterwards. I'm talking for years afterwards. I wondered what he'd done exactly and about how good it'd felt. I didn't talk about it and didn't ever try to touch myself (looking back, I wished I had). Seven years later, at 17, I got a boyfriend who touched me through my shorts and then took them off. And I felt the magic again. At that age, I still don't think I knew where my clitoris was (or what it was). But I was finally very motivated to learn.

—Suzanne, 33

JUST FOLLOWING ORDERS

The clitoris wants consistency. Why don't men know this? I can't tell you how many guys I've been with who don't take what I say literally. During sex I'd scream, "Right there, don't stop." Hearing this, these guys would somehow think, "If she likes that, wait until she sees this," and they'd do something completely different. I thought I was on track to have the best orgasm ever (or the best this week) and the guy would blow it.

After too many experiences like this, I decided to get this straightened out upfront. In the profile I posted on the Internet, I wrote, "If I say, right there, don't stop. I mean RIGHT THERE, DON'T STOP." You have to be clear. Men can get too excited in the moment. They want to please you, but they get carried away. The best time to give directions is when they're calm. My current boyfriend understands the meaning of "don't stop." Which makes him the best lover I've ever had.

—Dara, 36

A RUN TO THE FINISH

I got my clitoral hood pierced a couple years ago. I heard it would make sex more intensely pleasurable, and I thought, Why not? If it doesn't, I'll take the ring out. The piercing itself hurt—much more than when I had my ears done. I won't pretend it didn't. But I don't regret doing it.

A month after I got the new secret ring, I was in Las Vegas at a convention for work. I was late and tried to make the light across a broad street—six lanes of traffic—to get to the convention hotel. I was wearing very tight new jeans. Anyway, I start running and almost immediately I felt an orgasm coming on. My jeans were rubbing and the ring was moving against my clitoris. It was so strong and overwhelming I had to stop and put my hands on my knees and try to catch my breath. I knew I should keep going—I was still two lanes from the other side, and traffic was coming—but I was coming too. I couldn't move. I didn't even care. Can you believe that? It felt so good I didn't care if I was hit by a speeding car. Obviously, I lived to tell the tale. But, from that moment on, I've become an avid runner. And I avoid busy streets.

—Michelle, 30

SELF-SERVICE

You know how men say that no woman can give a better hand job than they can give themselves? Well, I feel that way about the clitoris. No man can make it feel as good as I can. I can't give them directions fast enough. How do you tell them how much pressure and when to move to more direct touching while you're thinking it? They're always going to be a little later than I want. That can be nice, but it's not as perfect. Don't get me wrong, I love having sex with my boyfriend. I like intercourse and he does a good job with oral sex and his hand, but he'll never be as good as me at getting me off.

—Roxanne, 28

Great Things Come (Ahem) in Small Packages

The clitoris is a little organ, but it's not as small as you probably think, you, and much of the world, including the medical establishment. In 1998, Helen O'Connell, M.D., a urological surgeon in Australia, went back to her textbooks and compared the anatomy drawings with the real women she'd operated on. She found that the anatomy diagrams for the female body—the ones she studied in medical school—had glaring defects and omissions. Like a few other doctors before her, she's proven that the clitoris is a much larger structure than the anatomy textbooks show. During my research, I found only two diagrams of the full clitoral structure done in this century. One was drawn in 1922 and published in the 1949 edition of *Atlas of Human Sex Anatomy.* Another was published in the *Journal of Pediatric Surgery* in 1970.

I knew that the diagrams I saw in the majority of medical textbooks were wrong just by looking at my own body. Thankfully, Dr. O'Connell and other researchers like her are finally correcting them.

Here's the truth: underneath the vulva folds, the clitoris *and its roots* look very much like a penis. The clitoris works very much the same way as the penis. Surprising? Yes. And too true to ignore. Dr. O'Connell explains that the clitoris "is a large structure that wraps around the vagina and the urethra. The external 'head' is attached to a 'body,' two 'arms,' and a mass of erectile tissue, called 'bulbs' which, like the penis, swell with blood when aroused."

To be clearer, the clitoris is shaped like a wishbone, the top of which is the clitoral glans or head that we can see under the hood when we look at ourselves. This external part of the clitoris can vary in size between a few millimeters to a half-inch. The clitoral head extends an inch or two into the body and then forks into two arms. The two arms of the wishbone are on average about four inches long. They straddle the urethra, running along under the skin where the labia are. From the roots to tip, the average clitoris measures roughly four to six inches long, close to the same size as the average penis.

For my Safina Salons, I decided to present what I learned in a quiz show format. I wanted to convey the details in a nonthreatening, cheerful way. I shout out a question and give the women in the room a chance to answer. If you get the answer right, you get a little prize (chocolate body paint, sample packets of lubrication, colored condoms). Women who don't have a clue aren't put on the spot and aren't made to feel stupid and inadequate. Stories flow naturally out of the quiz show format. It's proven to be one of the highlights of our Salons.

The Clitoris

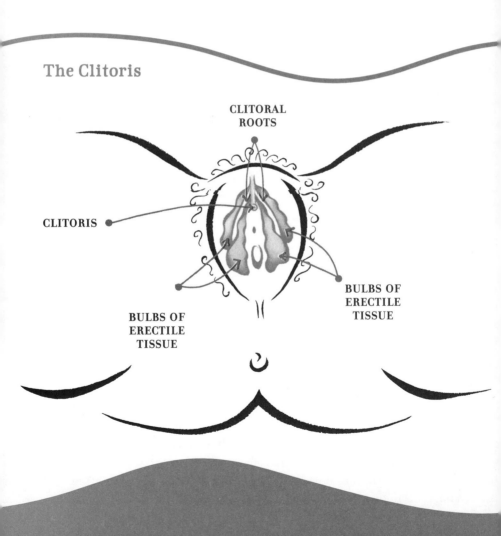

CLITORAL
ROOTS

CLITORIS

BULBS OF
ERECTILE
TISSUE

BULBS OF
ERECTILE
TISSUE

QUIZ SHOW QUESTION NO. 1:
What is the clitoris attached to?

SHORT ANSWER: Its roots.

LONG ANSWER: In most illustrations, the clitoris is drawn as a small red curve, which trails off inside the folds of skin near the top of the vulva. Any woman who's touched herself knows this couldn't be right. I can feel that my own clitoris is firmly attached and not some tiny floating pebble. The clitoris is, in fact, firmly attached, deeply rooted around the vulva like a wishbone. It has eighteen separate parts to it, which Rebecca Chalker, author of *The Clitoral Truth* outlines in her book. This may be a little inflated because she and the Feminist Women's Health Center count the blood vessels as separate parts. But no matter how you add it up, the clitoris is far more extensive than meets the eye.

QUIZ SHOW QUESTION NO. 2:
What's the difference between a clitoris and a penis?

SHORT ANSWER: The clitoris is MORE FUN.

LONG ANSWER: The penis and clitoris are more similar than different. The clitoris and penis have the same superstructure. Most of us know that all embryos start out female. Around the seventh or eighth week in utero, if the fetus is going to go male, the clitoris extends outside the body to become a penis. What might have become a vulva closes and develops into testicles.

The penis also houses the male urethra and is a sperm delivery system. So, while it's fun for play, the penis has serious work to do. The clitoris, on the other hand, has absolutely no practical purpose other than pleasure, and quite a bit of pleasure at that. It has four times as many nerve endings as the head of a penis, making it much more sensitive and responsive to the slightest stimulation.

The clitoris is the only human body part—male or female—that is solely for fun. Eve Ensler—creator of the renowned play *The Vagina Monologues*—has done a great job of pointing this out to thousands of people around the world. I'm trying to do my part too. We women are possessors of a tremendous source of pleasure, and yet so many of us discount it or ignore it. If men had clitorises, they'd never get their hands out of their pants. Doesn't the idea of penis envy seem absurd when you think about the sensitivity, specialization in pleasure, and compact neatness of the clitoris?

QUIZ SHOW QUESTION NO. 3:
Does clitoral size matter?

SHORT ANSWER (AS IT WERE): **No.**
LONG ANSWER: **Size is a hotly debated subject regarding penises.** But I've never heard a group of women (or men) swapping opinions on the pluses and minuses of having a big or small clitoris. Maybe if men couldn't compare with each other they wouldn't worry about it either. I was surprised, as you may be, to find out that clitoral size and shape varies just as widely as penis size. No two are alike. I found a book called *Feminalia* by Joani Blank that is a color photo collection of vulvas of all sizes and shapes. One after the next, page after page of photos, like any art book—but not the kind you want to take on the subway or bus. It is fascinating to behold the diversity. Some clitorises are visible, and some aren't anywhere to be seen at all. The variations of labia range from small and pink to large, dark, and almost ruffled. Most women are asymmetrical, and you can see that the terms "labia minora" and "labia majora" are misnomers. Just because they are "inner" lips doesn't mean that they are completely inside the "outer" lips. Very often the inner lips poke beyond the outer lips.

Brief digression: Last year, I met a plastic surgeon at a party in New York who is starting to do a brisk business in the field of labial surgery. This surgeon's clients want their labia altered to be symmetrical, tidy, and uniform. I was shocked at this unnecessary mutilation of the most intense bundle of nerve endings in the human body—all predicated on ignorance. These women must think they're abnormal and ugly. How would they know they aren't? How many other vulvas have these women seen? Airbrushed *Playboy* pictorials don't count.

Georgia O'Keefe, a leading member of the avant garde movement in the 1910s and 1920s, painted giant vulva-like flowers, with layers unfolding in shadows and light. Thinking about the vulva as an O'Keefe image is a very positive way to approach getting to know your own visually. It sounds very touchy-feely to suggest, but it is truly a good idea to take a look at your own vulva to see what's going on. Expect asymmetrical lips and several shades of color that change in front of your eyes. Don't fall into the trap of turning your vulva into yet another body part to obsess about negatively. Accept that you are normal and beautiful. There is no one way for a vulva to look.

Okay, digression over. Back to size variation. The average length of the external clitoris is a quarter of an inch. But the range runs from a few millimeters to an inch or more. Tanika, 24, attended a Safina Salon last year. "My boyfriend told me that I had a really long clit," she said. "It's about an inch long. I had no idea that all women didn't have one my size. Now I realize that my clitoris is an outie, just like a belly button. More of it is external than other women's. It works for me, and when I hear friends complaining about not being able to have an orgasm during sex, I figure I must be lucky. Because of my outie, I don't have a problem with that."

QUIZ SHOW QUESTION NO. 4: What is the right way to touch a clitoris?

SHORT ANSWER: Only you would know.

LONG ANSWER: **Women can learn a lot from men about sexual pleasure.** Basically, practice makes perfect. They know exactly what they like because they have hands-on experience. Men masturbate *a lot*. They've had years and years of practice. Why shouldn't women be as intimately aware of their clitorises as men are of their penises? We'd all have more fun. When you know yourself well, you can make sure your partner quickly learns what you like so he can have more fun by making you happy. Your ability to be open and to explore is both an intellectual and emotional choice. You have to want to do it, want to feel more, learn more, and trust more. Why would you let someone else have control of your pleasure? It's nice if men add to it, but make sure you don't turn over the driving to someone who's not in the car.

Now, let's get down to brass tacks. Just as there are variations in size, women differ in sensitivity. Some women are so sensitive that any direct contact is too intense and even painful. Other women need hard forearm-busting action to feel their best. See the box "Come On" below for some specific styles.

QUIZ SHOW QUESTION NO. 5: What happens to the clitoris during orgasm?

SHORT ANSWER: It spreads love and joy o'er this great land.

LONG ANSWER: **The very long answer, from the first tingle to the final explosion, a detailed moment-by-moment physiological and emotional breakdown, fifteen pages of sheer thrills and chills, can be found in chapter 4, "O Joy."**

Five Reasons Your
Vulva Is a Stranger

1. As a child, you were probably discouraged from touching or asking about that part of your body by adults.

2. Chances are, you might have associated the area with danger. Very early on, we're told to wipe front to back because of the possibility of infection. We hear language about the hymen "breaking" and are told about cramps and blood.

3. Comparing and talking about their penises is a rite of passage for boys. But girls never brag about their body parts, show them to each other, or talk about them. Somehow, girls get the idea not to mention it, as if showing interest is deviant.

4. Women and girls don't look at their own vulva. Men, if they could, would stare at their penises all day long. Women shun the area, finding it unattractive or offensive (although the shock of seeing it does die down).

5. If you have seen other vulvas, most likely they were airbrushed, photo-shopped images from soft-core porn magazines. Those aren't what real women look like. They're hairless, the colors have been altered, the shape has been changed, and blemishes have been erased. By comparison, you might think your own parts are abnormal. What's abnormal is making a photograph of a flesh and blood woman look like a plastic mannequin.

Come On

It's true that everyone is different. We don't wear the same clothes even though we all have arms, legs, and torsos, and we don't like to be touched the same way either. It took you years to figure out what you like to wear and you are probably still experimenting with shade and style. Experimenting with how you like to be touched is also ongoing adventure in trial and error. Put in the time and feel fabulous.

Orgasms are like snowflakes. The variations are endless. I have collected the following clitoral contact techniques from women in Safina Salons. If you have a favorite clitoral caress technique that isn't listed here, please e-mail me at comments@safina.com so that I can share the information with women at Salons. When it comes to touching, there are no rules of thumb. Clitoral advice: use lubricant so that you get sensations without the distracting friction, which can interrupt your dreaming mind. See "Lube Review" in chapter 6.

1. SPINNING.—**Have you ever taking a spinning class at the gym?** The best part of the class is when you take the tension off the bike and pedal as fast as you can. Around and around, smooth effortless motion. It's like flying. This is the best metaphor I can think of for the main technique women tell me they love. Use a lot of lubricant and start with big circles that pass over the clitoris as part of spinning around the top half of the vulva. Keep up continuous motion. Let yourself daydream. Slowly tighten the width of the circles towards the clitoris—or whatever part of the vulva wants attention. There's sensitive erectile tissue everywhere—below the clitoris near the urethra, at the entrance of the vagina—feel around. You're not limited to direct clitoral stimulation. Besides, that might not feel too good until you're warmed up. Take a spin around and find out what you prefer during different times of the month and when you're in different moods.

2. ELLIPTICALS.—**Ellipses or ovals are a favorite of many women who take the multifinger approach and who say that passing by the clitoris and coming back is the way to go.** This is a three fingered—or whole hand—rhythmic loop. Start with wide ellipses with a fixed point

as an anchor. Use the top of the clitoris as your anchor for a while, and then switch to the bottom side of the clitoris. For how low and wide to go with your ovals, think of the vaginal opening is six o'clock, go to six, then five, then seven. Expand your touches across the whole evening hour range. Try going fast or slow, or fast then slow.

3. THREE-LEGGED RACE.—**Placing your index and ring fingers on the sides of the vagina, use your middle finger directly on or around the clitoris.** Leave your wrist to rest on your pubic bone and slide your index and ring fingers up and down or in big circles involving the whole vulva. Your middle finger can either follow the other fingers' motion directly on or near the clitoris or it can make smaller circles or sliding motions inside the other two fingers. This approach is a little complicated and requires some coordination.

4. INSIDE AND OUT.—**Can be done manually or with the aid of vibrator(s).** With the hand: make a perfect C shape with your middle finger and thumb. Insert the middle finger into the vagina to touch the G-spot (see chapter 3 for specific help), and place your thumb on the clitoris. Make circles with your thumb, and press with your middle finger. With a sex aid: put a vibrator just inside the vagina, curved into the G-spot (see chapter 3) and put another one on or near the clitoris (or just get a vibrator that is designed to do both at once). Turn both vibrators on at a low speed at the beginning, and increase the speed at needed.

5. RUB-A-DUB.—**Fun in the tub.** Put the water on low pressure, just warmer than body temperature. If you have a hand-held showerhead, put it between your legs and see what your clitoris thinks of that. If you don't have a detachable showerhead, you can get a tube/hose-like gizmo at any hardware store. OR, you can lie down on the floor of the tub and position yourself (legs up on the shower wall) so that the water running out of the facet hits you just right. Something about the light but steady flow of water on or near the clitoris sends some women over the edge and into a whole new state of relaxed and energized. Waterproof vibrators are also fun and can give you something relaxing to do while you wait for your deep conditioner.

6. GETTING MORE C.— **Intercourse is nice**. Most women really like it but few have orgasms from it. Why not increase your chances by making sure the clitoris gets some attention during the act? Get on top and get your guy to squeeze his butt, raising his pubic bone. Put a pillow under him as well. Doing so will allow you to rub your clitoris against his pubic bone. Lean forward slightly, and you'll really feel the difference. Watching you love this will lead to new levels of fun for your guy, rocking his enthusiasm as well as the rest of him. Also, lend a hand (your or his) or add a vibrator to the mix. There's no reason intercourse should be a hands-free (or vibrator-free) activity.

7. TO THE LEFT.— **Do you find that one side of your clitoris is more intensely pleasurable than the other?** Steve and Vera Bodansky, authors of *The Extended Massive Orgasm*, think so, as do many women I've met. According to the Bodanskys, the upper left side of your clitoris (upper as in toward the ceiling) is the most sensitive. Please e-mail me if this is true for you (I have theories about left-handed vs. right-handed women).

8. THE SQUEEZE.— **Make a narrow V with your index and middle fingers and put the narrow part of the V on either side of the clitoris.** Then gently tug the vulva up and down towards your stomach and back down again. Progress to squeezing your V of fingers around the clitoris. Now put it all together, tugging and squeezing.

9. THE FLUTTER.— **Make another narrow V with your index and middle fingers.** Move the two fingers quickly in the opposite direction like kicking legs. That's what I mean by "flutter." Now place the narrow part of the V between the vulva folds so that your fingers are on either side of the clitoris. Flutter, flutter, flutter. Or, if it's too soon for that, work up to fluttering by squeezing, spinning, or other techniques first.

10. DELAYED GRATIFICATION.— **Holding off to have a bigger, more gratifying release when you finally come is more often done with another person than by masturbation.** . But you can do it by yourself to see if your orgasms really are more intense if you make yourself wait. There are two big tactics: (1) when you're about to come, stop what you're doing, wait for five beats, and then start again; and (2) don't zero in on the spot that most wants to be touched until you absolutely can't stand it anymore. Most of the time, however, with masturbation, the idea is to relieve stress quickly, getting rid of tension so you can sleep. But who knows, maybe you're the best tease of all.

Five Steps to Making Your Vulva Your Friend

1. Go to a bookstore and find a book like *Feminalia* by Joani Blank or *Sex for One* by Betty Dodson. Take a look at the photos or drawings of other women's parts. Notice the variations in color, size, and shape and the wide range of normal.

2. Get out the hand mirror. It sounds corny and it will feel silly, but you're an adult now. You don't have to worry that your mother or sister is going to burst into your room and catch you with the mirror between your legs. On a weekend morning, when the light is good, sit Indian-style on the bed and put a mirror in front of your vulva. Take a few seconds to get over the shock. Then look more carefully. Identify the parts (refer to the illustration on page 23). Notice if one lip is larger than the other, if your clitoris leans to the right or left. Get a clear sense of how you're put together.

3. After an initial superficial look, touch. Pull back the hood of the clitoris to expose more of the tip. Spread the vulva to see the entrance of the vagina. Lean back to see the perineum. (For more on the P-spot, see chapter 5). Notice how close or how far away the anus is to the vaginal opening.

4. You might be feeling something around now, especially after a general exploration of the clitoris. Good. When you're turned on, the whole area changes. Blood flow causes the lips to inflate, the wrinkles to smooth out. The clitoris becomes erect, like a penis. It gets harder, redder, bigger. Note these changes.

5. Since you're already down there, you might as well find the G-spot while you're at it. For a clear map, turn the page to chapter 3.

The Elusive G-Spot,
Located
at Last!

I found my G-spot in my senior year of college.
I didn't celebrate the discovery (I would have thrown a
party) because almost immediately after having found
it, I lost it, for seven years. I sort of hoped it would turn
up buried in the couch cushions or deep in a closet
somewhere. No sign of it though, no matter how hard
I looked. And believe me, I looked.

In the years I've been doing the Safina Salons, I've
learned that my story is not unique. What's even more
common, women who have never found their G-spot,
despite years of feverish hunting. Just as often, women
haven't bothered to look, assuming, since they'd never
felt it, it must not exist. Once I start talking about
the elusive spot, and assuring women that every female
has one, they all want to know the same thing: so
where the hell is it?

Of course they want to know. Who wouldn't want
to access yet another source of pleasure? Despite the
G-spot's media coverage and how the phrase is bandied
about as a universal truth, the area remains, sadly,
mysterious. If everyone who has ever said "G-spot"
knew where to find it, the world would be a very different
place, a happier place. I can tell you, since I've redis-
covered my G-spot and can find it as easily as the
back of my knee, life has gotten a whole lot brighter.
I am duty-bound to spread the joy.

Is that it?
I think that might be it.
Or not.

The first time I tapped into my G-spot, I was uninformed and clueless. I didn't have a name for the sensation, but I sure knew something different was going on. I was seeing John. He was one of my study partners' roommates. He had dark hair and dark eyes and a silly laugh, and he was so hot-blooded he wore shorts in the winter and a light short jacket and really was warm enough. He always convinced me to get on top, which hadn't been my favorite position. But from my perch, I saw that John was having a great time and was in no rush. I relaxed and started to enjoy myself. I slid around and explored how it felt to move this way and that. John had all the time in the world for me to enjoy myself. He wasn't the kind of guy who drove relentlessly, unswervingly, to orgasm. Sex was a journey for him.

I was a happy passenger. While I was on top, John would do this thing where he arched his back and held my legs in place. We'd stay like that for a long time. Sensations would surface, like none I'd felt before. Sex with him was a welcomed new experience. I had whole-body orgasms with him, ones that started somewhere deep inside me and could clear my sinuses. I wasn't really sure where they came from, nor did I care. I just wanted more of them. I believed that the amazing fresh feelings were because of John, the shape of his penis, his technique. I didn't realize that sex with him was so great because together we were stimulating a place in me that hadn't been reached before.

Well, John and I broke up. If only relationships could be based solely on fantastic sex and last. Sigh. The worst part was that when he walked out the door and disappeared from my life, so did my G-spot. It lay dormant, waiting impatiently, with excruciating frustration, until I met Paul. He was prematurely gray, five years my senior, smart with a quick wit and the kind of confidence that makes women swoon. That confidence came to bed with us. He was always in charge sexually, even if it was to put me in charge of him. He also liked me to get on top.

And then—hello!—I had that same overwhelming feeling, the one I never thought I'd have again. Just like with John, I didn't know where it was coming from exactly. I just wanted the feeling to continue, for a few minutes, or into next week. He shifted, and the feeling ebbed. I yelled, "Don't move!" I may have scared him a little, but he listened. I wiggled around, finding the feeling again. For fear of losing it, I decided to study it, right then. I rocked, moving him against me to hit the epicenter of the feeling. I tested it, investigating the boundaries of it, and realized that the sensation was radiating from a particular area. And then it hit me hard: this feeling is not from him, it's from me. Sure, his penis was hitting the right place in me. But the spot itself, that wonderful spot, was all mine.

In the seven years since my introduction to this spot, I'd read about the G-spot and was left wondering if that was what I'd felt so long ago. As I sat on Paul, shifting and rolling against him, I thought to myself, "G-spot, my old friend, we meet again." I was so glad to hit the jackpot that I stayed there for what seemed like hours, getting to know the feeling intimately, in vivid detail. Poor Paul couldn't hold back anymore and that was that.

I was so thrilled, I didn't care it had ended. I'd taken the time and had the presence of mind (barely) to get a good handle on where to find my G-spot. Nowadays, with all the practice I've had, I could be a tour guide to my G-spot. I could (do) find it in the dark and I've still never seen it. I have a mental signpost with big arrows pointing directly at it. As well I should.

As well you should too. You too can get to know your own body and all the ways you can feel great. Isn't that better than drifting about aimlessly, hoping to stumble across something powerful by luck or accident? Just think of the relief—for both you and your partner—if you can describe explicitly how to hit the spot. He'll be so happy, you'll be surprised. It doesn't matter that you had to tell him where to go; he'll glow with pride at having arrived there. There are, of course, times in life when we find ourselves between partners. With or without partners, it's wise to know yourself and how to feel good on your own.

So Where the Hell Is It?

Patience, patience. Before I get into the nitty-gritty of finding your G-spot (I'll practically draw a map, a really good one, better than the ones you've seen elsewhere that use anatomically incorrect drawings—just bear with me for one tiny bit), I want to touch on why the G-spot is still so shrouded in mystery for most women.

REASON NUMBER ONE that the G-spot is the holy grail of sex: **Women don't talk about it with each other.**

That's why I said earlier that I feel duty bound to describe G-spotting in detail. Women seem to stop short of divulging the most pertinent sexual information to each other. When I'd initially tapped the G-spot in college, I didn't tell anyone about it. Sure, I gave the nonspecific report to my friends, as in, "John is so hot in bed," etc. I did not, however, announce that he'd hit a place inside me that I'd never felt and desperately wanted to feel again. When I knew enough to give it a name, I didn't call my friends and announce that I'd won the jackpot. I kept the news to myself. Until I started Safina, I hadn't had a single balls-out conversation about finding the G-spot. No one ever asked me, so I never told. The whole subject never came up among my girl friends, even if it was mentioned in the women's magazines we all read from time to time. The men I dated, meanwhile, wanted to know all about it.

It wasn't that I didn't want to tell my friends about the G-spot or to hear their stories. It didn't even cross my mind to do so. Sex talk was always vague and nonspecific. None of my friends told me if or when they found their G-spots; we never debated where it was or talked about the possibility that men have one (they do; see chapter 5 for more information). Now graphic descriptive tendencies differ from woman to woman, from group to group. But, again, not to flaunt the evidence of the Safina Salons, I've heard hundreds and hundreds of women, from their early 20s to their late 50s, confirm my belief that women may dish about sex, but they don't rush to serve up explicit details.

It's funny that women can go on forever describing protein intake or the syllable-by-syllable tone fluctuations used by a potential love interest on the phone. We can go on and on about food and love, but sex gets the silent treatment. Well, not completely silent. We have Monica Lewinsky and *Sex and the City* to thank for that. Women can certainly talk about the sexual exploits of public and televised people, but they can't seem to talk about their own. Again, I mean in detail. You can see the cursory throwing around of the words "sex" and "orgasm" on nearly any prime-time TV show. But you sure won't hear Grace tell Will that she bought herself a keen new vibrator and has finally stimulated the G-spot to the point of female ejaculation. No, no. Our popular culture has come a long way since the frigid-fearing '6os, but we're not quite ready to be that frank about vaginas in our lives let alone on prime time.

You may be cringing right now at reading the very word "vagina" and all the explicit detail in this book so far. It's a "private" part, not for mass discussion, right? Women have told me that discussing the G-spot is still "too personal" or "too much information." That is one thing I want my Salons to change for women—their comfort level with talking about sex. Men can talk about their penises and not cringe. They can admit to masturbation and show a woman how to please them. We women should have the same freedoms and the same healthy attitude. It's sad that we don't. Seems a shame, doesn't it?

This is why we, in lieu of woman-to-woman discussion, go to magazines for directions to the mystical ganglia. Which brings me to: REASON NUMBER TWO that the G-spot is the best kept secret of womankind: **Even with a map it's hard to find, and most directions are way off.**

Let's start with the most basic illustration of the female reproductive system, one we all know. Many of us could draw it from memory. I'm talking about the diagram that goes with the instructions inside a tampon box. You know, the side view, one leg raised, tampon poised to enter. Most of us saw it for the first time at the age of 12, and it left an indelible impression. Let me make one thing perfectly clear: THE TAMPON BOX DIAGRAM IS INACCURATE.

It's misleading. You know this already. Your vagina isn't the shape of a test tube turned upside down, gaping open and angled straight toward your tailbone. But this is what we believe our bodies would look like if we were sawed in half and became transparent. I think this is why so many women, including myself, struggled with inserting a tampon at first. The diagram didn't show a big muscle to push past. It didn't show the hook inward. My early tampon experiences were a misery of agonizing frustration and painful half-insertion. Only when I figured out that you had to push past that initial, undiagrammed partition between the inside and the outside was I able to successfully insert a tampon.

Naturally, when women go looking for the G-spot, they're surprised to learn that there's a big bump of muscle that curves inward toward their abdominal-side vaginal wall, instead of the smooth, straight tube pictured in the tampon diagram. Confused? No wonder! You were expecting a straight shot, and the road has a hairpin curve. That curve is about one third of the way in and is the key to finding the G-spot.

When I started the Safina Salons, I wanted to find an anatomically correct illustration to show to women. I went to the biggest textbook store in town and spent an entire day going through every medical textbook I could find. I thought I'd find a few illustrations to choose from that would clearly show the G-spot and the region as I understood it, and then I could just show women where to find the G-spot, and other points of interest.

I ended up buying the three most popular medical textbooks. I took all three books home, scanned the diagrams, enlarged them, and took them to my gynecologist. My doctor couldn't believe what trouble I'd gone to when I showed them to her. I explained to her that I was determined to find the best illustration possible for the Salons. I expressed my concern, saying that I thought each of the diagrams was inaccurate. She said, "Everyone knows the diagrams are all wrong. The best medical illustrations were done by Frank H. Netter in the 1930s, and could stand updating."

The main thing that was missing from these diagrams (and the diagram in the tampon instructions) is that the vagina is drawn in the unobstructed test tube style. My gynecologist explained that these illustrations are based on drawings from cross sections of cadavers (which of course don't have tight muscles). She showed me the three-dimensional clear plastic model of the female pelvis and said, "You think the diagram is bad, look at this." We stared at the disproportionate model with its pre-pubescent hips and short fat vagina that led to a large solid-colored uterus and big fallopian tubes. "It's completely disproportionate within itself even if it's not supposed to be at a 1:1 scale," she said. The G-spot is unmarked in the textbook illustrations and the plastic model. I theorized to my doctor that "the G-spot is excluded from medical education because it doesn't get sick." She considered that and agreed. Most doctors are only interested in parts that cause problems. The only problem with the G-spot, however, is the lack of informational material about it.

Look at the illustration on the next page. This is gynecologist approved, with all parts clearly marked and shapes and sizes proportionate to scale. Compare it with the famous tampon diagram. Like night and day.

Two last quick points about the great unsolved mystery of the G-spot and then down to the business of what, and where, it is. REASON NUMBER THREE for the bafflement: **The G-spot vanishes!** Not by magic. The tissue that makes up the G-spot is erectile. Just like a penis, or a clitoris, or nipples. When you get sexually excited, they get hard, swollen, bigger, full of blood. Same thing with the G-spot. Just like an erection, it is only there if the mood is right. The G-spot is tactilely invisible and undetectable unless you're hot and bothered. When you are aroused, it swells, inflates, and gets a ridgy texture.

With this in mind, I'm not at all suggesting you throw this book aside and hunker down to find your G-spot with the same determination you might start a first novel or run a marathon. The G-spot doesn't respond to that kind of pressure. Think of it as shy. Don't plow in, demanding its presence. It'll vanish on you.

Finally, REASON NUMBER FOUR: **The G-spot sensation is often misunderstood.**

Stimulation of the G-spot can easily be confused with the feeling that you need to pee. There's a simple anatomical reason for this, which I'll get to in a minute. When a partner finds a woman's G-spot, she may experience a very pleasurable feeling completely intertwined with the sensation that she must excuse herself immediately and rush to the bathroom. In reaction to this sensation, women tense up, stop thinking of the pleasure and sensation, and focus only on not having an accident.

In Safina Salons, it's always a satisfying moment when I describe this sensation to a group of women and then hear many of them say, "I've felt that." Understanding is the first step toward openness to new experiences. I tell the women that if they're getting the have-to-pee sensation, they're on the right track, not to seize with fear, and to let the feeling wash over them. They look up at me with relief and gratitude, eager to leave the Salon and go home to their partners to try it out. So, without further ado, let's get to the matter at hand.

The G-Spot

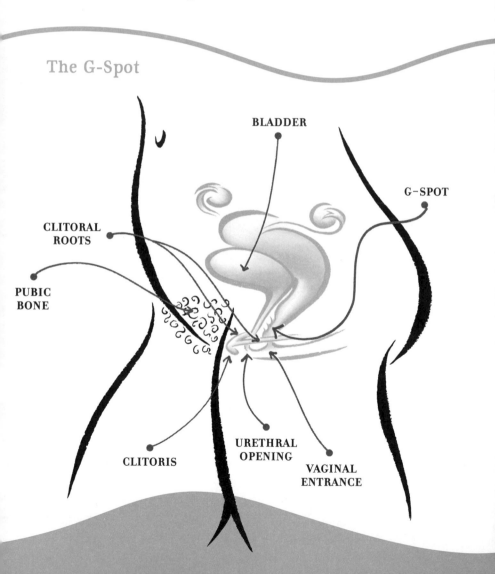

BLADDER

G-SPOT

CLITORAL
ROOTS

PUBIC
BONE

CLITORIS

URETHRAL
OPENING

VAGINAL
ENTRANCE

The Nerve

Some basic anatomical information: when you put your finger into your vagina as you curve along the abdominal-side front wall, you can feel ridges. What you're feeling through the vaginal wall is the protective tissue wrapped like insulation around the urethra (that's a tube connected to your bladder out of which you urinate). That protective tissue, the insulation, is erectile tissue and is filled with nerve endings. When you're turned on, that tissue becomes enlarged and richly sensitive. The G-spot is part of this band of sensitive tissue. Light bulbs must be going off: this is why stimulation of the G-spot—actually, stimulation of the urethral wall—can be uncomfortable or confused with the sensation of having to urinate.

The spot itself is really an area, a dense patch of ridgy texture that varies in size from woman to woman. Just as the cervix varies in size from as small as a silver dollar to as large as a small pancake, your G-spot might vary in size from a nickel to a half-dollar. You may also find it only to realize that it's not very sensitive or that it's not your favorite sensation, but you might as well know that for sure instead of wondering. It could be that it's your favorite place in the world . . .

The Search Party Begins

Break out the rubber gloves! Kidding. But actually, before you start the expedition deep into the core of yourself, you will want to have some lubrication at hand. Lubrication is another topic that goes undiscussed between women. There is a mistaken notion that it should be unnecessary. Lubrication is as necessary as hand cream. You might not want to use it every day, but it's great to have around and really, you can never have enough lubrication. If you've never tried it, you'll see it adds to your fun and feels great. I recommend Liquid Silk, but K-Y will do in a pinch. Don't use household products though. Use real lubricant to avoid upsetting the natural balance of your body. With a partner or alone, this search will be fruitless unless you're in the right frame of mind (the

G-spot just won't be there). So go pee (to avoid anxiety about that), and then get yourself excited in whatever way you prefer.

Now, locate your pubic bone. Imagine you're wearing jeans, and press down on where the base of the zipper would be. Feel that hard bone? It's lower than you might have thought. Most women, when searching for the pubic bone, start pressing in middle of their pelvis and have to work their way down. The pubic bone is about one-third of the way into your vagina. The bottom one-third of your vagina is where most of the nerve endings and sensation are concentrated (probably so you don't die of pain when you have a baby and your cervix has to open up). THE G-SPOT IS DIRECTLY BEHIND THE PUBIC BONE. **That's marker number one.**

Next, acquaint yourself with the pubococcygeus muscle (henceforth, PC muscle). This is easy. Once again, think tampon insertion. When women first give this a go, the wall of resistance that they have to pop through to get the tampon far enough into the vagina often troubles them. That wall of resistance is the PC muscle. You can feel it at the entrance of the vagina, but it stretches all across your bottom from your pubic bone to your tailbone like a hammock. Without it, you couldn't keep a tampon in place, you'd be incontinent (in fact, one way to find the PC muscle is to stop your urine stream), and you wouldn't have powerful contractions during orgasm. It's jam-packed with nerve endings from the clitoris to the anus. To understand the G-spot, you must visualize the PC muscle. Picture the vagina as if it were a drawstring bag. When you pull a drawstring bag shut, there's still a small opening, right? Imagine that is the opening of the vagina. The cinched part is your PC muscle. Just past the cinched part, there's extra room. And that is where to find it. THE G-SPOT IS JUST BEYOND THE TIGHT RING OF MUSCLE AT THE VAGINAL ENTRANCE. **That is marker number two.**

Moving along, knowing where to look is well and good, but you need a method for getting there. Take your hand and put it in the air and motion for someone to come over to you—the come-here motion we all know well. Turn your hand sideways while you're in the middle of doing the "come here" motion and notice the steep curve of your index finger, the backwards "C" shape. If you inserted your fingers into your vagina and put them back into that same position, you'd be behind your pelvic bone and right in your G-spot area. Be sure to move your fingers around, pressing on your abdominal-side vaginal wall. Keep them curved into the C–shape, but try some circular motions to find the hotspot(s) of your own G-area. If you want, although you might laugh and totally ruin the mood, say, "Come here, G-spot" to attract its attention while making the motion inside.

Locate Your G-Spot

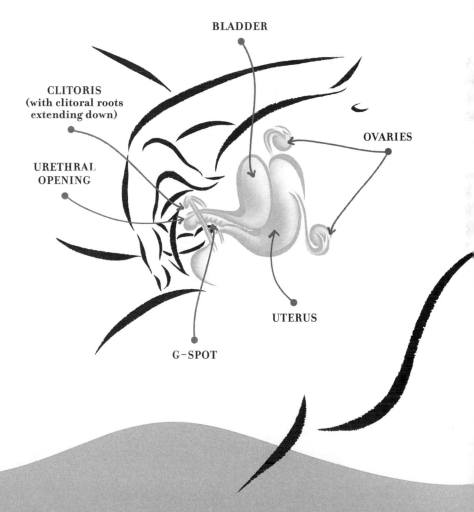

BLADDER

CLITORIS
(with clitoral roots
extending down)

OVARIES

URETHRAL
OPENING

UTERUS

G-SPOT

To Recap

1. You can do this alone or with a partner.

2. Lubrication is key.

3. Eliminate fears: make sure you pee beforehand.

4. You won't find it unless you're already turned on (because it won't be there).

5. The G-spot is behind the pubic bone.

6. It is just beyond the PC muscles on the abdominal side of your vaginal wall.

7. You can access it by making the come-here motion with your fingers.

8. This is supposed to be a fun exploration, not a sweaty, overly determined hell-bent quest. Relax and poke around. You might strike gold.

The G-Spot in Position

Before trying to hit a perfect G with intercourse, I strongly advise you find it first with your own hands, your partner's hands, or any of the wide selection of ergonomically curved G-spotter vibrators/wands (we call them Sexories at Safina). Vibrators will probably help you find it faster because they will tease the tissue into becoming erect. When you know your G-spot as well as you know the location of your nose, you can guide someone else to it. The worst thing to do is to give someone directions and have them get lost. Be sure of the way there yourself.

Reminder: Tell your partner not to do a pressing-a-button motion. The same motions that work on the clitoris are a good idea.

If you want to stimulate the G-spot during intercourse, your partner doesn't have to be an expert at finding it with his penis. You can shift position so that he's hitting it. Think of it like geometry: how can he be angled so that he's dragging along the front/abdominal-side wall of the vagina? Based on what I've heard in Safina Salons, MISSIONARY POSITION IS THE WORST FOR G-SPOTTING FOR MOST WOMEN. **Here are two positions that are better:**

1. **Typically, the position is referred to as "doggie style," but the term seems so insulting.** Of course, we need to suspend judgment and have fun, but somehow, equating yourself with a dog taints the whole thing. And I love dogs! But still, I don't want to be one. So let's refer to it as the Position Formerly Known as Doggie Style, or Admiring the Sheets. For G-spotting, Admiring the Sheets is the way to go. The penis enters at a downward angle; think 45 degrees, in and down. You can control the angle by adjusting with your elbows or moving your head closer or farther from the bed.

2. **Topside. Good G-spot contact here.** The man is on his back while you straddle and face him. Instead of going at it like a man would (bouncing up and down), slide in a circular motion as well as and back and forth, towards his feet. This makes anatomical sense, and you may very well enjoy it because by sliding around, you'll be stimulating the clitoris as you go. Bouncing ignores this epicenter of nerves. By angling your body towards his feet, the penis can push into the G-spot.

What the G-Spot Can Do

So you've found the G-spot, and you enjoy the sensation of it. Many women who have orgasms with some G-spot stimulation find them to be deeper, more intense, and more satisfying. But that is just the beginning of hot G-spot action. Consider the wet spot. That circle of dampness one often finds after sex, which seems just too big to blame solely on the man's ejaculate (only a tablespoon or two of fluid at most).

So, whence the wetness? As you know, the general topic of sex goes largely undiscussed, and certainly no one wants to chat casually about excessive bodily fluids. I know there are hundreds and possibly hundreds of thousands of women who believe that, at some point, they have wet the bed. Some are convinced they've peed in it, others just know they've flooded it, and still others marvel at that occasional wet spot, wondering how it got there. No one, of course, wants to sleep on it. Generally speaking, the wet spot is considered a bad thing. It's spoken of shamefully, as in, "look what I did," instead of the accomplishment it is, as in, "look what I can do."

THE FLUID IS THE RELEASE OF G-SPOT-TRIGGERED FEMALE EJACULATION.

I don't love the term "female ejaculation." I find it clinical and unsexy. The only slang I've heard—"gush" or "squirt"—is worse. Unbeknownst to most people, women can ejaculate a fluid like men do. So similar, in fact, that the liquid is called "prostatic fluid." The female ejaculate comes from near the urethra, from the paraurethral glands on either side of the urethral opening and in the urethral sponge (or G-spot), but it is not urine, nor does it contain sperm (obviously). It is extremely similar to sugary mix that is produced by the prostate in men (which the sperm then joins before coming out as semen). According to Dr. Beverly Whipple and Dr. John D. Perry, authors of *The G-Spot*, about 40 percent of women experience female ejaculation and most women have the potential to ejaculate (my guess is that many are losing these orgasms to the fear of peeing). Since female anatomy education in school is confined to the ovaries, fallopian tubes, and uterus, many women (you'd be surprised) don't know where their urethral opening

I thought women peed from the clitoris the way men pee from their penis. After the Safina Salon I went to, I went home and got out a mirror, and I still couldn't really see the urethral opening. So I held up the mirror while I peed to see where it came from. I felt really silly, but I didn't want to stay so clueless. I'm 39 years old, and I didn't know how my body pees and holding up the mirror I could clearly see it was like half an inch from the clitoris.

is in relation to the vaginal or anal openings, let alone the glands around the urethral opening.

Some women experience the female ejaculation as a series of spurts. For others the ejaculate fluid just leaks out at some point during sex without much fanfare. Many have experienced both. The quantity varies also from one woman to the next and from one romp to the next. It is possible to soak most of the bed, or it can be not much more than the usual amount of lubrication one always makes. It can happen quickly, or it can take over an hour of direct G-spot stimulation to occur. However, the important thing to realize about female ejaculation is that it's completely normal—and desirable. Women who've experienced it say it feels great. With all G-spot related activity, the best advice is to relax, explore, and do it for the sake of fun. Don't think of yourself as inadequate if you find it and lose it or do or don't have an ejaculation. The G-spot is merely one more avenue of pleasure to investigate. So do.

Salon Secrets

I've certainly produced a lot of fluid, but one night, my boyfriend and I had been having intercourse for a long time, and I was getting to the point of wanting to stop. And then, I felt this sensation building deep inside. I can't say where exactly it came from, but I'd never felt it before. My vaginal muscles started to contract, but not in the way they usually do during orgasm. And then, I felt four distinct squirts of fluid jet out of me. Like I was pumping them out, but I had no control over it. I didn't have my typical orgasm when it happened either, but the sensation was deeply satisfying, as if I had this stuff inside me and it needed to get out. My boyfriend was just as shocked as I was. We stopped and looked at the bed. There was a huge wet spot, as big as a dinner plate. I said that it had never happened to me before. He said it hadn't happened for him with another woman either. Nor has it happened since for me. But I'm ever hopeful!

Important Dates
in G-Spot History

1.8 million years ago Early woman evolves from apes, with all anatomical parts fully formed, including the G-spot.

1913 *The Frigidity of the Female Sex* is published in Berlin by Alfred Adler, Austrian psychiatrist and creator of the system of Individual Psychology; first to describe the "inferiority complex."

1934 American psychoanalyst Edmund Bergler studied marriage and judged 70-80% of women are frigid – as defined by the inability to have a vaginal orgasm.

1950 Ernest Gräfenberg, M.D., says that Freud is wrong, that women are not frigid if they don't orgasm during intercourse (a widely held belief at the time). He tests the theory that women have nerves on the anterior vaginal wall (something Kinsey disagreed with). Gräfenberg's tests showed, " An erotic zone always could be demonstrated on the anterior wall of the vagina along the course of the urethra." Hence, Gräfenberg "discovers" said spot, and it gets named after him.

1983 Beverly Whipple, Ph.D., et. al, write *The G-Spot*, a best-selling book that details the area and introduces "female ejaculation" to the masses.

1988 I meet John and find my G-spot. Didn't know what it was, but liked it.

Late 1988 Lose John, and my G-spot. Missed the G-spot much more.

1995 Meet Paul, and rediscover my G-spot. Cling tightly to it, more tightly than to Paul.

O Joy

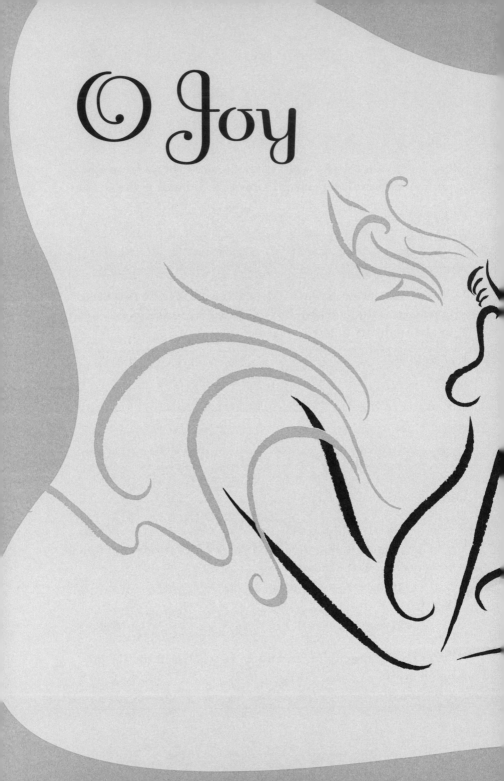

Chapter 4

Here's a little riddle for you:

What can be learned well but not summoned at will? What happens in your muscles but starts in your mind? What always makes you feel wonderful but can both wake you up and put you to sleep?

Anyone who's seen the movie *When Harry Met Sally* remembers the famous deli scene when Meg Ryan gives Billy Crystal an impromptu performance of faking an orgasm. I was amazed at the perfect crescendo of her simulated climax, and a little embarrassed too, squirming in my theater seat just as Billy Crystal was at the table. While watching that scene, I thought about the sound of an orgasm for the first time and realized that everyone must make pretty much the same noises. A universal sound of abandon had to be echoing in bedrooms all over the world, for real, or as in this case, as in an Oscar-caliber performance. And why, I wondered, was this such a surprise for me and for the millions of men who were shocked by that scene? Surely men had some idea that women could fake orgasms.

ANSWER: ORGASMS

Orgasm Expertise

You can blink on purpose, but the involuntary reflex of blinking every ten seconds guarantees a continually lubricated eye. Orgasm, also an involuntary muscle contraction, is not a blink. Orgasms, for one, don't just happen every ten seconds, nor are they something we don't realize we're doing until we think about it. For many women, they don't happen easily, by rote, or at all.

You have to learn how to have one (which can be a lot harder than learning how to *fake* one). We get this knowledge filtered through the media—movies, books, music—but mainly we learn how to have orgasms by hands-on experience with a partner or alone. It is not, I repeat, something that just happens for most women without the process of learning how to do it. Despite this, many Safina Salon goers have asked me why we need to learn about sex on purpose.

One of our first customers, Angela, a 40-something no-nonsense woman from a middle-class suburb in New Jersey, attended a Safina Salon out of curiosity. When she realized there was going to be lots of discussion instead of passive entertainment, she said, "I'm not comfortable talking about sex and I don't see why we need to." After that she sat back quietly listening to me and her friends talk about all sorts of things. When I was saying goodbye to her she said, "I've been having sex for about twenty years more or less but I learned a lot tonight that I'm looking forward to trying." Weeks later she gave me a call and said she was sorry she'd been so negative when she first met me. "After hearing my friends talk I think maybe I just need to be a little more open-minded. I think I'd kind of given up on the idea of having orgasms and I figured it was just me." The information gathered at the salon—anatomy lessons, sexual tips from friends, introduction to toys—did the trick. She said she'd been figuring out what worked for her since the Salon, that she was having more orgasms now, and that that was putting her "in the mood" a lot more often. "I'm just feeling great. Plus my husband is thrilled with my interest. We've been having a ball together, so I just want to say thank you!" Now, of course, she's hungry for knowledge.

Why doesn't he just know what to do?

The guy I'm dating has no clue what I like. But I'm afraid to move, or guide his hand. He might think I'm a slut, or be intimidated if I do anything. I keep hoping that he'll catch on by the noises I make. I tried to make it clear what wasn't working but he cannot take the hint. I thought it would get better over time, but it hasn't. And now, after all this time, if I did say something, he might feel betrayed. Now I'm stuck. —*Amanda, 32*

Amanda has been faking for so long, she can't even remember what sex is like without faking. This is the worst possible pattern to fall into, but Amanda's situation is fairly common. A 2002 survey by *Cosmopolitan Magazine* found that two-thirds of the participants had faked an orgasm. The two biggest reasons women aren't having orgasms with their partners are:

1. THEY ARE AFRAID TO GIVE THEIR PARTNER HELPFUL SUGGESTIONS.
2. THEY ARE AFRAID TO TOUCH THEMSELVES DURING SEX.

In both cases, what ruins their fun is fear.

Amanda, and thousands of women like her, get into bed afraid of what will go wrong, instead of excited about what will go right. She's terrified about being greedy for pleasure. She's afraid that her partner will think she's a pervert or slut if she tells him what to do or (God forbid) shows him by touching herself; that even the slightest suggestion that he isn't hitting the right spot will make him cower, shrink, or cry like a baby; that the male ego is an eggshell; or that he'll resent her desire for satisfaction and think of her as demanding and selfish, whether it's for more time and less pressure or for him to do a certain thing.

I may sound combative, but I don't mean to. I know women are under a lot of pressure to get a man and to keep him. I have a mother who wants grandchildren. I understand exactly what it feels like to want to hold onto a man and to be afraid of losing him. But I also know that sacrificing your sexual satisfaction will not keep him around, nor will faking to make him think he's satisfying you. I, for one, would rather be single forever (sorry, Mom) if the relationship I was in didn't give my orgasms equal time. And I certainly don't want to marry a man with whom I don't feel comfortable enough to tell him or show him what works for me. Imagine a lifetime of faking orgasms, trying to sleep afterward, being too unsatisfied to rest, and even sneaking into the bathroom after sex to masturbate. Lying, deceiving, and only hurting yourself. Ecch. What a dismal way to live.

Consider the alternative: great orgasms, open communication, mutual satisfaction, and deeper connection. Of course, a new man doesn't know your body's ins and outs right away, but he wants to be told what he can do for you. He's watching you to see what effect this move or that has on you. He doesn't expect you to like all of them. He's working on trial and error and would appreciate any guidance you can give. Believe me: he wants to be good at this. He wants to send you deep into a red-hot sea of lust and pleasure. He *lives* for it! A turned-on woman is the ultimate turn-on for a man. You could blow him for five hours straight, and he won't get as excited by it as he would from watching and feeling you come against his hand, lips, or penis or with the help of one of Safina's very lovely accessories for your lust life (more on that later).

Every now and then you might come across (as it were) a guy who does know what to do. That's nice (hell, it's amazing!), but just because his skills give you a free pass from having to communicate your needs doesn't mean you should keep your mouth shut. Even if he's a genius in bed, if you talk more about what feels good, you'll both discover new tricks and add to your repertoire.

Practice Makes Perfect

One of the reasons women are so often frustrated by men's ineptitude is because they believe men know more about sex than women. Wrong. Well, let me take that back. Men do know themselves better than most women know themselves. Men start masturbating earlier. They aren't taught to avoid or fear their own body parts like many women are. Unlike most women I've talked to, men aren't embarrassed that they are experienced masturbators. Almost all adult men know that spanking the monkey and having orgasms is normal and that *not* masturbating is weird and wrong. They feel no shame for normal body maintenance— and that's really what orgasms are for men. Get up in the morning, brush the teeth, check the gut in the mirror, and jerk off into the toilet. Or into a tissue. Or in the shower. Men will have an orgasm whenever there's a little free time before or after work. They do, *because they can.*

Meanwhile, women often have guilt, shame, and discomfort about masturbation. Our society is really weird about sex, as I've mentioned before, especially about women's bodies. We're obsessed and yet we're silent and restrictive. Your negative views around masturbation go back into childhood: every time you were told not to touch yourself, every time you were discouraged from asking about it. Boys, on the other hand, grew up encouraged to masturbate by their friends and even their fathers who told them it was normal. While you spent your youth avoiding the area, worried about your hymen, afraid of getting pregnant, and trying to be a normal nice girl, boys were spending their free time becoming experts on their own orgasms. Seventy-five percent of boys hear about masturbating before they ever try it. When did you first hear about it? Did you ever hear about it now from an actual person (putting magazines and books aside for a moment)? Ninety percent of American boys have 2.3 orgasms a week by the time they are 15. Twenty-three percent of girls have one orgasm per week by the time they are 15. Plenty of women have their first orgasm after college. We aren't slow learners. We just shirked practice.

As grown women, we continue to be uptight and proud of it. As we grow up, we think in terms of being a good girl or a bad girl and that thinking stays with us. What does being a "good girl" do for you once you're out of high school? It's a childish concept. But now we're adults. Let's stop thinking in terms of good and bad and try these questions instead: Am I happy? Am I satisfied? Am I healthy?

Despite the fact that good sex is the key to good health and the glue in any monogamous relationship, women still frequently dismiss the importance of their own physical pleasure as if it didn't matter. Meg Ryan's Sally character explained faking an orgasm as an easy way to make the man feel good. And what about Sally feeling good? That wasn't even an issue.

Women can have orgasms as easily as men. To do so, they have to learn their own responses as well as men. Men have a head (hand?) start with masturbating, but women can catch up. For women to become accomplished, we must first think differently, starting with the language of it. Every woman hates the word "masturbate" as much as I do. It's almost as horrible as "horny." It took me years to be able to say it out loud. I still don't like the sound of it, despite the fact I say it many times during a Salon. It's just a word, a superficial thing. But, in hating to use the word, women are inhibited in our thinking, our ability to talk about it and, yes, even do it.

Men have a million euphemisms. They're cheerful, creative, silly, and so often about animals. Spank the monkey, drain the snake, choke the chicken. They have some good gender-neutral euphemisms: "master of my domain" from *Seinfeld* is still one of my favorites. Then there's my friend Carey's favorite, "taking a solo flight," or the new age-intoned "moving my chi." The only female-exclusive euphemism I know that isn't offensive is "polishing the pearl." My friend and coauthor Val likes "taking some private time" or "going bowling."

So let's talk about one of life's great pleasures without any negative judgment attached. Pick a euphemism. Any euphemism. Whatever works for you.

The Solo Flight

There's a mistaken notion that solo flights are only for when we're not in a relationship. Back to *When Harry Met Sally.* Remember Sally confronting one of her many boyfriends about his masturbation during their relationship? She whined, "Aren't I enough for you?" while looking incredibly hurt and feeling horrible about herself. He said, "Oh, come on, don't tell me you don't masturbate anymore since we got together." "I don't," she insisted back, as though this were a virtue. She went to Harry and told him how upset she was and how wrong her boyfriend was, and Harry said, "Everyone does it. It's normal." And he was right. It is normal. Not just for men but for everyone.

Sally's idea that being in a relationship changes things is part of the female tendency to put pressure on their relationships to satisfy every need. The dream that a girl grows up with is that someday she'll meet a man and he'll take care of her in every way she needs and she'll take care of him. A very nice idea. And it is true that, in a healthy relationship, you can take care of him and he can take care of you. But you are and always will be in charge of your orgasms. You should have as many as you can with and without the guy you love.

Solo flights take the pressure off the relationship in the same way you blow off steam bitching to your girlfriend about his leaving socks on the floor. With a solo flight, you don't have to be in the same place at the same time or in the same mood. Expecting him to be totally responsible for your satisfaction is like saying he's the only friend you'll ever need. It's an unreasonable pressure, and it won't make either of you happy. Always keep your friends *and* your solo flights. Encourage your man to do the same. That's healthy independence. No one can live up to the pressure of completely satisfying the needs of another person. That's unhealthy dependence. Who wants to be on the receiving or giving end of that?

Masters and Johnson have noted that many women have their most intense orgasms when alone. I've heard similar claims at Safina Salons. Maybe that's due to the lack of distractions, pressures, and worries that often accompany sex with a partner. Katisha, 31, a mother of one, told a Salon group, "I know when to go faster, or slower. I don't have to hope he'll listen to my breathing and I don't have to worry about what he's thinking. I'm the best I've ever had."

AN INTENSE ORGASM IS A GIFT TO GIVE YOURSELF THAT ALWAYS FITS, AND IT WILL CHANGE YOUR OUTLOOK AS WELL AS YOUR LOOKS. **Try it on. Here are a few things to keep in mind before going it alone:**

1. **Just as you allot time to do your nails, pluck your eyebrows, and apply makeup, you must give adequate time to a solo flight.** It should be a relaxing sojourn. Joy can't be rushed. As with everything else you do to take care of yourself, the benefits of a solo flight will show themselves in your appearance. You will look better, and you'll feel fabulous.

2. **Explore.** Try lots of different tempos, fingers, strokes, vibrators, dildos, lubricants, etc. Switch between hands, go towards the clitoris, around it, the sides of it, try something inside while moving around the outside at the same time. Don't just find something you like. Find everything you like! (Regarding lubricants and vibrators, see chapter 7 for useful dos and don'ts.)

3. **Let your mind wander.** Fantasies will come and go. Good. Don't pressure yourself over what images or storylines are right. Daydreams really don't have anything to do with real life so don't judge yourself. If one image isn't working, move on to something else.

4. **Enjoy the journey.** Like a long bath, a facial, or a massage, a solo flight is for relaxation and good mind/body maintenance. Relax and enjoy every second, and your body will follow. Let go of any goal. Orgasms come out of nowhere when you're having fun (like all good things), but they can't be forced. If you chase your orgasm, it will hide. They are stubborn like that.

I don't want anything for myself, I just want to make you happy.

As recently as a 1983, 80 percent of surveyed women said that they didn't feel cheated if they didn't have an orgasm during sex because it was more important that their partners were pleased. (I bet that if you polled the men being referred to here, they would say that it's important that both they and their partners have an orgasm. If only the woman had one, I bet 100 percent of the men would feel cheated.)

This statistic is another indication that women aren't comfortable talking about sex. Sure, we can talk about relationships until we're blue in the face. But sex? We aren't comfortable talking to our friends about it, and so we definitely aren't comfortable talking to the men we're involved with. The result of silence? Women decide to be selfless to avoid having to communicate. "I just want him to enjoy himself. I enjoy being with him. I don't need to have an orgasm." Noble? Admirable? I don't think so. You're not just cheating yourself, you're lying to this guy you supposedly care about.

Let's set the record straight here: your orgasm matters. It matters just as much or more than his because it's yours. I've heard women say that it's sometimes fun to have sex even if they didn't have an orgasm during it. That's nice. It happens, certainly. But it's still a letdown, isn't it? There is nothing selfless about not having an orgasm. You don't get extra points for denying yourself, and chances are, your guy feels lousy for being the only one who got off. In the movie, Sally tells Harry some women must have faked with him at some point. He doesn't believe it. Sally shows how well she can fake and wins the argument. But she's losing out in life. Sexual frustration is not fun, no matter how well you fake it.

Performance Anxiety

Performance anxiety is something we think of as a male problem. After all, he has to get it up and then make sure it doesn't go down before it should. Failure to stay hard is often joked about, a source of shame. Less so now, in the age of Viagra, but still, men have pressures we don't.

Which isn't to say we have none. Women have performance anxiety too. The pressure to have an orgasm inhibits the orgasm. He's pumping away, saying, "Come on, go ahead, now, do it" and a whole slew of other things that mean, "You have my permission to hurry up" or "I'm waiting and ready." Not to be a male apologist, but most men aren't aware that this is pressuring you. If they remember saying anything, they think they were cheering you on. This is why communication is so important. If he knew his "cheering" was making you tense, he'd stop it.

Often this pressure is on top of the fact that women haven't had enough solo flights to really know what works for them. If you don't know what works, you can't do it or tell him to do it, and all the while he's making you feel like you'd better hurry up or you'll miss the boat. It's no wonder so many women practice their acting skills. In case I haven't made my point by now, here it is one more time for posterity: faking is the worst kind of lying. It's addictive. It becomes habit because you don't know how to get yourself out of this predicament once you get yourself in. Once you've faked, you've programmed him to do whatever he was doing over and over again in the future. Like all bad habits, it's best not to start. If you've already established the bad pattern, you can start over. It's worth it.

Tell him you're reading this great sex book.

To transition away from faking, or to instruct your guy on all you've learned during your solo flights (try at least ten before bringing up the following with your partner), introduce the subject of hot, new moves by blaming me. Say, "I've been reading a book by this scx expert, and I thought we'd try some new ideas." He'll be all over that. I guarantee it. Then take a step-by-step approach.

1. **Tell him from the start that you want to do only new moves tonight and not fall back on what you usually do.**

2. **If he forgets, and starts up with the old way, slowly disengage and remind him that tonight is all about the new.**

3. **Be honest and say, "Well, that new move isn't working for me," or, "Now that's a discovery worth marking on a map."**

4. **Sex is serious fun. Keep your mood light and your body will feel it and be more relaxed.**

Sex Is Like Shopping

You don't look good in every piece of clothing you pick up, but does that make you give up and just go without? Lots of things you try won't be to your liking, but that's how you find out what you do like.

You try on a lot of clothes before you find the perfect outfit. Also, depending on the time of the month, something looks great on one day and looks terrible on another day. It's the same with sex. Different days require different approaches. Experiment with moves, speeds, positions, and accessories.

Sometimes, shopping is goal oriented ("I need a new coat"), but you wind up buying something unexpected ("no good coats, but I got killer shoes"). Don't go into a sexual encounter with a goal in mind. Just enjoy the expedition.

So What Is an Orgasm?

Let's talk about what really happens physiologically from beginning to end with an orgasm. Since most of us have gotten a sparse education in our basic anatomy, it's hard to know what our bodies are going through when we come. It's not self-evident. Nothing about the body is. I've been eating all my life, and I'm still learning about how to do that better.

Unfortunately, science has a long way to go to pinning down the female orgasm. There hasn't been a ton of research on it, and medical reasoning is slow to evolve from times past when women were the weaker sex and their frustrations were considered ailments Many researchers fear that their study in the area of female sexuality won't garner them respect. There aren't a lot of grants or funding available to them. They have to battle conventional wisdom, which is a tough sell. But then again, the subject of nutrition continues to baffle researchers. Ten years ago, we were told bacon was bad. Now bacon is good. Or is it?

Regarding sex research, we'll start shortly after the start of modern thinking (Alfred Kinsey's post World War II surveys of real sex behavior in America vs. cultural ideals kicked this era off). In 1966, Doctors William Masters and Virginia Johnson divided sexual response into four distinct phases, charting the first detailed study of the orgasm (male and female). Since then, we've learned that the four stages aren't quite as distinct. Furthermore, the research only examines muscle contractions and the flow of blood (toward and away from the genitals). That said, the stages do hold up. They are excitement, plateau, orgasm, and resolution.

What the stages model doesn't take into account is everything else that goes on during sex. The mental (self-esteem, body image, religious issues, shifts in consciousness) and emotional factors (love, connection, the whole range of feeling) that go beyond the purely physical. And on the physical front, an orgasm affects more of your body than your genital area. A whopper could potentially clear up your sinuses, make you less depressed, release muscle tension, and help you sleep. But we'll get to that. First, the stage-by-stage breakdown:

1. I'M SO EXCITED AND I JUST CAN'T HIDE IT.

The excitement phase is a blur of fantasies, urges, and sensation.

It starts in your mind and then it takes hold in your body. Your breathing changes, the vagina starts lubricating itself, and at least twelve distinct hormones and natural chemicals are released into your blood and brain. Blood flow rushes to your vulva and causes erectile tissue to swell. The clitoris becomes erect. It literally pokes out from its foreskin hood; its roots stiffen and elongate. In baboons, the female genital area becomes so swollen and wet that part of her body becomes, literally, a puffy red flag, waving the male of the species to come on over and get some action. If human males could be like baboons and take a moment to look for physiological changes in their partners' bodies, they'd see clearly why foreplay is crucial for a woman's enjoyment of sex. As we all know, readiness is everything.

2. ON A SHELF OF EXCITEMENT.

The plateau phase is a deepening of excitement and sexual tension.

It could be called excitement part 2. Nipples stiffen and breasts swell (they can increase in size by up to 25 percent for women who haven't had children; mothers show less of an increase, if at all). Blood continues to rush to the genitals. All that extra fluid causes the vaginal opening to tighten by about 30 percent; the labia puff up and spread out and go from pink to dark red. Masters and Johnson noticed that if the color change doesn't happen, a woman won't have an orgasm. The vagina elongates, and the deepest two-thirds of the vaginal alley balloons to nearly twice its normal width. Vaginal lubrication decreases at this point, and the clitoris, still erect, sneaks back under its hood and is often too sensitive to touch directly. Just touching the vulva near the clitoris at this point can be plenty. Also, 50–70 percent of women experience a "sex flush" on their chests and face as a result of blood moving to the surface of the skin (that's why so many romance novels talk about skin feeling like it's on fire, scorched, scalding, etc.). Heart rate increases and breathing quickens. This phase gets the body completely ready for intercourse and is necessary for any kind of orgasm.

3. OOOORGASM.

Whether or not an orgasm is a predictable crescendo once it starts, it often comes out of nowhere.

Sometimes quickly, sometimes not as quickly as you'd like. All women describe their orgasms differently, and like snowflakes, no two are exactly the same. They may feel centrally located, or diffuse throughout the body. They can start in your head, and shoot down to your toes. No matter how or where you feel it, any orgasm is right on the money. There is no such thing as a bad one.

Orgasms require a bizarre blend of concentration and relaxation. Or maybe you could call that absolute focus—pinpoint mental acuity on physical sensation. Orgasms are outside the realm of control. Trying to look composed when you have one is a sure-fire way not to get there. Orgasms can embarrass us. They are almost too primitive, reminding us that we are animals.

The low down: physiologically speaking, an orgasm is a spasm of the vagina's muscle floor, which runs through your clitoris as well as your anus (from pubic bone to tail bone). Waves of spasms flow through the entire uterus as well. I've heard pregnant women talk about ninth-month orgasms as being especially intense because their uteruses are so huge. A number of feel-good hormones flood the brain as well, notably oxytocin, which is known as the "love hormone," and endorphins, the chemicals that are associated with "runner's high."

According to a study of women in the United Kingdom, the average orgasm lasts twenty seconds. Try counting to twenty. Takes a while, no? Other studies say six to ten seconds. Again, like clitoral size and vaginal shape, there is a range of length and intensity from woman to woman, orgasm to orgasm. I've had orgasms that were as brief as a sneeze, others that seemed to last all day, and into the evening (but were probably just fifteen seconds). The number of spasms for an average orgasm tends to be between three and seven rhythmic spasms, but I have a friend who says she's counted well into the twenties (how she could count and still be having one is amazing to me). The spasms come at a rate of about one per second. Muscles throughout the body can spasm and tense to rigidity during orgasm; brain wave monitoring shows how an orgasm plays out in a woman's head as well.

On average, women need eight minutes of *direct* clitoral stimulation to reach orgasm. That is only an average. Many women need much more time to come, depending on the state of arousal and lots of other factors. Some women don't need direct contact; others don't need any clitoral contact (there really are some women who orgasm just from nipple play). Women are also able to have brain-only orgasms, climaxing in their sleep, the female equivalent of a man's wet dream. Alfred Kinsey found that 37 percent of the women he studied had experienced sex dreams with orgasm by the age of 45 and the frequency stayed constant from adolescence through 50 years old. The highest instance and frequency of male orgasms during sleep occurred during their teens (70 percent) and then dropped off significantly from their 30s onward.

All women are physically capable of having multiple orgasms, defined as one orgasm spilling into another and another, without a refractory period between. According to Betty Dodson, author of *Sex for One* and the high priestess of orgasm training for women, the key to multiples is breathing through an orgasm (not holding your breath, which is typical). Easier said than done, of course. Learning to breathe during orgasm takes practice. Dodson also mentions that orgasms range in intensity and that perhaps multiples are a pileup of small blips, as opposed to a huge bang. Timothy Leary claimed to have seen a woman on LSD have a hundred orgasms in a row. Sex researchers have documented women having fifty plus, and even back in 1953 (when this must have been a really taboo subject) 14 percent of Kinsey's female subjects reported having multiple orgasms regularly. There's probably no limit to how many you can have. The book *Extended Massive Orgasm* purports to teach women how to keep orgasms coming for an hour. For the purposes of this book, I'd like to concentrate on making sure my readers have at least one every time they have sex. A modest goal perhaps, but you've got to start at the beginning, and go (I mean, *come*) from there. See the sidebar later in this chapter on how to multiply your fun with multiple orgasms.

Compared with men, women are more orgasmic. Men come and all the blood flows away from their penises, making them soft. They have to wait a few minutes at least to get hard again. Women don't have the same refractory period. The excess blood in our genitals doesn't rush away as quickly and completely as in men's. We don't have to wait, and therefore we are ready to go again immediately. It's ironic that women have been considered less sexual than men when, biologically, we are engineered for greater pleasure.

A brief caveat: the last thing I want to do is to make any woman feel inadequate if she takes longer than eight minutes to come, or never has multiples, or needs to take a long break between sessions before she can come again. Some of the most sexually self-actualized women I know don't tend to have more than one orgasm in the same day. Sometimes a clitoris is just way too sensitive after orgasm to be touched again for an hour. My desire is to simply let women know what's going on with other women so that we can all come again and come often, however we each see fit.

If you've never had an orgasm, you may wonder what it feels like. The French refer to it as "le petit mort"—the little death. While it might sound a little gruesome, it does encompass the intense feeling—the stopping of time, the blocking out of place, thoughts, anything but sensation, and the losing of oneself in the moment. Or maybe they mean that you have to die a little to get a taste of heaven on earth.

Masters and Johnson collected descriptions from their female subjects about the sensation. Here's the consensus, as they recorded it: it starts with "a momentary sense of suspension, quickly followed by an intensely pleasurable feeling that usually begins at the clitoris and rapidly spreads throughout the pelvis. The physical sensations of the genitals are often described as warm, electric, or tingly, and these usually spread through the body. Finally, most women feel muscle contractions in their vagina or lower pelvis, often described as 'pelvic throbbing.'"

Anaïs Nin, erotic short story author and bohemian extraordinaire, describes the experience in her poetic and risqué diaries using phrases like "a fiery and icy liqueur through the body," "the pleasure of a gentler wave," "electric flesh arrows," "a rainbow of color," "a foam of music." She was trippy and mad for them, saying each day demands one.

Resolution—winding down once it's all over—doesn't have to happen right after orgasm for women.

As I mentioned above, if sexual stimulation continues, a woman can experience additional orgasms. But once stimulation stops, postorgasm(s), the body returns to its normal relaxed state. The uterus and vagina revert back to their normal placement. The breasts and vulva go back to their normal size and color but may remain sensitive for a little while. Breathing and heart rate settle down. The sex flush fades. If an orgasm hasn't occurred, there will be a feeling of heaviness and pelvic discomfort. Remember men's complaints of "blue balls?" Well there's no gender bias in discomfort when it comes to getting all worked up and not having a release. Blood is trapped in the pelvic organs and needs to be dissipated by orgasmic muscle contractions; everything is in a heightened state and waiting.

Eventually, even without an orgasm, the body will calm and the blood will dissipate. The discomfort, however, takes time to resolve. Frustration isn't fun. If you think you're being selfish by wanting to have an orgasm after your guy is done, think again.

How to Multiply Your Fun

While multiple orgasms are a lot of fun to aim for, don't ruin the orgasms you already have by pressuring yourself to have more. The key to multiple orgasms is to surf a wave of pleasure. So catch a wave and keep on riding it instead of waiting for it to break. That's very different from what most of us do. We tend to do what men do: build up to a giant single orgasm and then they rest. Often they just drop off to sleep. Unlike men though, we have other options. Most women aren't aware of this. And why should they be? It's not like we have multiple orgasmic role models, but now we do have some research. If you haven't had any or many multiple orgasms, consider the following:

1. **When you feel an orgasm start to build, keep breathing.** Think about the orgasms you've had. Do you tend to hold your breath?

Most of us do. Deprivation of oxygen to the brain heightens orgasm. Excited, erratic, shallow breathing at the point of orgasm is practically instinctual. But this breath holding makes it difficult to keep going from one orgasm to another. First, your brain demands oxygen, so after you come, the blood flows out of the genitals and back to the brain. But to come, you need the blood in the genitals. Keep your breathing normal and you won't divert blood flow back to the brain.

2. **As you keep breathing through an orgasm you might feel like you're losing orgasm momentum.** Keep in mind that this is only the first wave of pleasure and don't expect it to feel like one big event.

3. **Visualize multiple orgasms as a drive into the mountains. First there are the foothills and then the bigger peaks.** Go toward them without any expectation and wander around. Don't try to get to the top of a big peak. It's all about the journey, not the destination. A big peak can rise up behind any foothill, and a series of foothills can stretch on for a long, fabulous trip. Don't try to force anything. After all, not finishing is the goal.

4. **Multiple orgasms require time, the absence of pressure and lots of lubricant** (you can never have too much lubricant anyway, but in this situation it keeps things flowing nicely).

5. **As I mentioned earlier, orgasms often come out of nowhere.** Concentrate on what feels good to get the first one.

6. **Try to stay in the moment, which will take you onto the next one.** Keep breathing through and let go of the goal of having any orgasm at all. Try this with or without a partner and notice the differences in the two situations. Be a keen observer of your own pleasure.

7. **Once you experience going from one orgasm to the next you will, more and more often.**

8. **Don't judge yourself or your orgasms.** Multiple orgasms are great, but so is one strong explosive one and so is the simple feeling of massage all around the clitoris all on its own. Don't pressure yourself to achieve anything and you'll have more of everything.

Sexual Frustration through History

ABOUT 70 PERCENT OF WOMEN CAN'T HAVE AN ORGASM THROUGH INTERCOURSE ALONE. Not surprising to accomplished solo flyers, 90 percent of women who masturbate do so by stimulating their clitoris exclusively. Only 10 percent of women stimulate their vagina while masturbating, and even they usually stimulate their clitoris at the same time. Despite all this expertise, many people (of both genders) are under the impression that a woman should be able to get off through standard intercourse and to come at the same instant as her partner.

If you believe that, you probably think Prince Charming will be arriving shortly with a glass slipper in your size. As I mentioned in chapter 2, this female orgasm myth was embedded in our culture by men like Sigmund Freud, whose three essays on sexuality (published in 1905) misinformed generations about the nature of the female orgasm. His belief was that the clitoral orgasm is immature and should be transferred to vaginal orgasm, that is, one had during intercourse once a girl hits puberty (or really once women have started having sex with men). Written like this, doesn't it sound silly? What's wrong with a clitoral orgasm? Why should we need to transfer anything except to conform to irrational male beliefs? Freud's theories on the female orgasm, by and large, are ridiculed nowadays, but medical experts throughout history have labeled women's sexuality as various forms of illness—he wasn't the first, but he had an enormous impact on the twentieth century. All the way back to the fourth century B.C. until 1952 (half a century *after* Freud's early fame), women who didn't orgasm during intercourse were "diagnosed" with hysteria and "cured" by being brought to orgasm manually by a doctor. Women's inability to have an orgasm through intercourse was considered a deficiency and an illness.

To my ears, this sounds like a ploy to make women feel bad about themselves, to get money out of them by pathologizing their natural needs, and to make the male feel better about himself. And it definitely sounds like a way to take advantage of them while charging them under the pretext of practicing medicine. Imagine going to a doctor today and he tells you he's going to molest you and then take your money because you're a sick, sick woman. You'd be on the phone to the police in three seconds flat. Back then, however, the job of treating (read, getting off) hysterical women was odious. No one wanted to do it, least of all the husbands, which is why the medical establishment took over at great profit. Pleasing a woman is a dirty job, but someone had to do it. It wasn't until 1952 that the American Medical Association made a declaration to its members that hysteria is not really an ailment and ended a long span of time during which vibrators were "medical devices."

Even though men knew women didn't have orgasms from penetrative sex, doing anything manually or orally for the woman just wasn't done. They believed a woman's pleasure should mirror the three phases of male pleasure:

1. GETTING READY FOR INTERCOURSE,
2. INTERCOURSE, AND
3. RELAXING AFTER INTERCOURSE.

This thinking lingers, even now. Consider this: is it "real sex" if your partner penetrates you and comes, but you don't? Is it "real sex" if you give him a blowjob or jerk him off? Is it "real sex" if he goes down on you and nothing more? Expanding the definition of real sex to revolve around a woman's orgasm or to include oral and manual sex without penetration is still a hard sell. Bill Clinton didn't view his hummer from Monica as "real sex." For the most part, the nation agreed.

Medieval writers actually thought that women experienced pleasure by receiving male semen and believed nothing else was required to satisfy them. Semen was promoted as salubrious for women, so much so that contraceptive barriers were discouraged despite sexually transmitted disease and the life-and-death risks of childbirth.

Cultural taboos around masturbation made this situation even more horrible. A solo flight was considered immoral, a danger to women's health, and a cause of insanity (ironic, isn't it, that NOT masturbating drove these poor, frustrated women over the edge). More crucially, the men of that age believed that masturbation could lead to a lack of interest in intercourse and infertility. Furthermore, as men wrote in medical journals through the seventeenth and eighteenth centuries, woman who actually enjoyed sex were considered nymphomaniacs who were likely to cheat on their husbands, thereby threatening the concept of monogamy, the framework of the family, and the entire construct of a civilized society. Women were doomed if they didn't get off and under suspicion if they did.

The diagnosis of hysteria ended in the middle of the twentieth century, not that long ago, only to be replaced with "frigidity" (a concern that went back to the early Freud days as well), which is defined as a lack of interest in intercourse or coldness to a husband's advances. Frigidity was treated with muscle relaxants, hypnosis, and psychotherapy. In 1910, up to 75 percent of "civilized" women were thought be frigid (see how the numbers remain creepily consistent?). Turn-of-the-century radicals spoke out and suggested that hysteria and frigidity were both due to brutish treatment by husbands. But these dissidents were thought of as a bunch of crazies. As recently as the 1960s, doctors were actively discouraging men from satisfying their wives. Dr. Alexander Lowen, author of the 1965 book *Love and Orgasm*, was a student of Wilhelm Reich's, who was looking into the orgasmic response and repression of sexuality, and Dr. Lowen had been writing on it himself since the early 1940s. By 1965, he knew and was clear in his writing that women needed direct clitoral stimulation to orgasm, but he made it clear that he empathized with the men at that time who thought that there was no good time to do this. He said that most men feel that bringing a woman to "climax through direct clitoral stimulation is a burden." Before intercourse was a bad time because the man could lose his erection doing all that hard labor, during intercourse he could use a hand on the woman but then his penetrative rhythms might be disrupted, and after intercourse he wouldn't be able to relax and the act would "be deprived of its mutual quality." So even with doctors who understood women's anatomy and sexual response, the male-centric focus of sex persevered.

The diagnosis of "frigidity" also persevered, but its definition shifted slowly in the 1970s and 1980s from the inability to have a "vaginal orgasm" to "absence or lack of sexual pleasure sometimes to the extent of lack of orgasm." Still, there were people writing about frigidity and cures in medical literature even in the late 1970s. *Frigidity: What You Should Know about Its Cure with Hypnosis* is one example, published in 1979, that was aimed at doctors and that was actually all about a new hypnosis technique to cure the same old illness as described in 1909. It didn't get a very positive review in the *Journal of Sex* in 1980, so times have changed, but change sure does take a long time.

It wasn't until the 1970s that women's sexual health and their need for orgasms their own way were taken seriously, and it had everything to do with women speaking up for themselves. That shift took place within my lifetime—and probably yours too. Its origins go back to Margaret Sanger, who promoted contraception and women's health in the 1910s; it was was fueled by Betty Friedan's 1963 book *The Feminine Mystique* among others and helped along by the formation of the National Organization for Women in 1966. But the first *Our Bodies, Ourselves* in 1970 was clearly one of the key moments in the shift toward acceptance of women's health and sexuality from their own perspective. This book helped thousands of women learn about their own bodies and start living in them differently.

Now, thirty-five years later, we still haven't completely let go of the orgasm-through-intercourse-alone concept, as if simultaneous orgasm were the ultimate in sexual bliss. It is a romantic idea, and it can be done—especially if you add clitoral stimulation to intercourse. Remember though, we aren't shaped the same way as men and our sexual response is different and perfectly normal. The motions that send them over aren't the same motions that consistently send us. Their pace is different— they move through excitement and plateau much faster than we do. Plus, they usually control the movements during intercourse as they approach their orgasm. Instead of obsessing over simultaneous orgasm, just enjoy yourself and enjoy each other and have orgasms however your body wants them.

Calling All Orgasms

No one is sure of how many different types of orgasms there are, but everyone knows that not all orgasms are equal. Some are faster, lighter, deeper, longer, more intense, full body, localized, more emotional, or more physical. Lou Paget, in her book *The Big O*, lists ten distinct types of female orgasm: clitoral, vaginal, cervical, G-spot, urethral opening, anal, blended/fusion, zone (some area of the body), fantasy alone, breast/nipple, and mouth (an orgasm from a kiss).

Well, here's what I think. Many people think both vaginal and cervical orgasms involve some clitoral or G-spot friction. Considering the layout of the vagina, how do you touch the cervix or the anterior wall of the vagina without touching the clitoral roots or G-spot? I have no clue. "Blended" means more than one of these areas stimulated at once, which seems like double counting. "Zone" means anywhere not listed in the other areas. This can happen, a great kiss on the neck for example. I've heard stories from women about this, but it's not exactly a daily occurrence. "Fantasy-" induced orgasm is clearly possible as evidenced by orgasm dreams and the fact that all of these orgasms are in the mind no matter where we attribute them on the body. In 1992, Dr. Beverly Whipple, author of *The G-Spot* and president-elect of the American Association of Sex Educators, Counselors and Therapists, found that orgasms without any touch, from fantasy, are physically experienced as though touch-induced. Since all orgasms do happen in the mind, I suppose having one from a kiss (or "mouth orgasm" according to Paget) is possible. I am skeptical that 20 percent of all people have experienced one. If only it were that easy. Maybe we're kissing the wrong people.

What all this really shows it that sex really is in your head. Whipple says that orgasm originating from the G-spot area uses different sensory pathways than clitoral orgasms. They are distinct and deeper. There's a lot of research to be done still on how the nerves are connected to our various parts and our various orgasms. We all have a lot of exploring to do. You might have a spot on your thigh that will send you over the top (the T-spot?). Being touched on your neck might push you into spasms of ecstasy (the N-spot?).

No matter how it's spelled, here are the ABCs of O: if you have one or a hundred spots that push you over the edge, congratulations. You don't need ten different kinds of orgasms. You only need one to be happy, healthy, fulfilled, and content.

Salon Secrets

I didn't think it was possible to have an orgasm without the standard making out and lots of rubbing. But I had an orgasm once when my boyfriend lightly touched me through my pants. It was his first move but I'd gotten so worked up in a very sexy conversation with him, I exploded the minute he touched me.

You know, there's a spot on my neck that my husband finds. There's something about the way he breathes on it, the way he kisses it. If he does that at the same time as he's touching my clitoris, I have orgasms that leave me seeing spots.

When I was 24, I had the most amazing experience that I would like to have again. My boyfriend was using two hands on me. One on the clitoris and the other swirling around inside me in circles near my cervix I think. I have never come like that before or since. It was the combination of his intensity and my mood I guess. I felt the orgasm through my whole pelvis. I think I felt it into my hipbones.

Come into Good Health

ORGASMS AND EVEN SIMPLE SEXUAL AROUSAL ARE NATURE'S PLEASURE PANACEA. SO LET YOUR LIBIDO LOOSE. COMING AGAIN, AND OFTEN, CAN HELP YOU:

1. **Sleep better.** Many people sleep more deeply and restfully after satisfying lovemaking or a solo flight. In the relaxing afterglow you may be able to let go of distracting thoughts. Being able to stop thinking has been known to help overcome insomnia.

2. **Feel less stress.** People having frequent sex often report that they handle stress better. The profound relaxation that typically follows lovemaking, with orgasm for women and ejaculation and/or orgasm for men, may be one of the few times people actually allow themselves to completely let go, surrender, and relax.

3. **Boost your immune system.** A 1999 study involving college students found that the levels of immunoglobulin, a microbe-fighting antibody, in students who engaged in intercourse once or twice a week were 30 percent higher than in those who were abstinent. Also, sex might make you actually heal faster when you're injured. Researchers in Sweden have found that oxytocin, one of the hormones released during sexual arousal, healed sores on lab rats twice as fast compared with the nonaroused levels of oxytocin in the blood.

4. **Reduce depression, anxiety, and even physical pain.** Hormones that are released during sexual excitement and orgasm can lower levels of "arthritic pain, whiplash pain and headache pain," according to Dr. Whipple. Just being sexually excited causes various hormones to surge into the blood. Two of these hormones in particular that seem to have a very positive health impact are oxytocin and DHEA:

    * Oxytocin, what's been described as a "feel-good" hormone, surges up to five times as high as its normal blood level during orgasm and is responsible for helping us forge close emotional

bonds (it's often known as the cuddle hormone); but it also regulates body temperature and blood pressure and speeds wound healing and relieves pain (from headaches to cramps and overall body aches). The release of oxytocin triggers the release of endorphins (hormone-like chemicals that are also natural painkillers and depression fighters). Orgasms boost levels of the female sex hormone estrogen, which also adds to mood improvement and helps ease premenstrual symptoms, according to University of Virginia researchers.

✳ DHEA, a steroid hormone derived from cholesterol and produced by the adrenal cortex, is important for a healthy libido and has been linked to reducing the risk of heart disease (seems ironic that it is derived from cholesterol, doesn't it?). DHEA is the hormone that proves that the more sex you have, the more you'll want to have it. In a DHEA supplement study reported in the New England Journal of Medicine in 1999 women reported "significant increases in frequency of sexual thoughts, degree of sexual interest, level of mental satisfaction with sex, and their level of physical sexual satisfaction." They also reported improvements in depression and feelings of anxiety. "Just before orgasm and ejaculation, DHEA spikes to levels three to five times higher than usual," says Theresa Crenshaw, M.D., author of *The Alchemy of Love and Lust*.

5. **Strengthen your heart.** Sex helps increase blood flow to your brain and to all other organs of your body. All that deep breathing and increased heart rate saturate organs and muscles with fresh oxygen and hormones. As the used blood is removed, waste products that cause fatigue and even illness are carried away. "Regular lovemaking can also increase a woman's estrogen level, protect her heart and keep her vaginal tissues more supple," states clinical psychologist Karen Donahey, Ph.D., Director of the Sex and Marital Therapy Program at Northwestern University Medical Center. Also, DHEA has been found to actually strengthen the heart muscle after a heart attack, which is why doctors recommend sex as soon as a heart attack victim is strong enough. It seems to me that the old myth about sex being

bad before the big game can be dispelled once and for all now that so many athletes find that DHEA supplements improve their performance. They might as well have sex before the big game!

6. **Maintain good sexual health.**Use it or lose it. Good sexual health has to be maintained. "Women who abstain from sex run some risks," according to recent article in Forbes Magazine on the necessity of sex. Dr. Winch, a gynecologist from Nevada, says one of the risks in postmenopausal women is vaginal atrophy. He has a middle-aged patient who, after three years without any sexual activity, is a prime example. "The opening of her vagina is narrowing from disuse. It's a condition that can lead to dysparenia, or pain associated with intercourse. I told her, 'Look, you'd better buy a vibrator or you're going to lose function there.'" If she did, she might find that the oxytocin and DHEA released in her system would lift her libido.

7. **Live longer.** A ten-year study of middle-aged men in Wales studied found the mortality risk was 50 percent lower in men with a high frequency of orgasm than in men with a low frequency of orgasm. Decreasing the risk of cancer in particular seems to be one of the big side effects of sex. In Australia, one study showed that the men who ejaculated more than five times a week were a third less likely to get prostate cancer in particular. Also, frequent sexual activity has been tied to lower risk of breast cancer in women. The reasons aren't completely understood yet, but the theory is that oxytocin and the sex hormones estrogen and testosterone have some role in cell signaling and cell division.

The positive benefits of sex—from depression to cancer to pain (which clearly straddles the body and mind)—show just how intertwined the body and mind are. Dr. Ronald Glaser, Director of the Institute of Behavioral Medicine Research at Ohio State University says, "The associations [between sex and longer life] are out there, so there has to be an explanation for it." Apparently, the advances in imaging techniques plus a constantly improved understanding of the biochemistry of arousal is helping researchers to start narrowing in on how it all really works. However it works on a cell level, the health benefits are clear: getting all hot and bothered and doing something about it is good for you.

P-Spotting

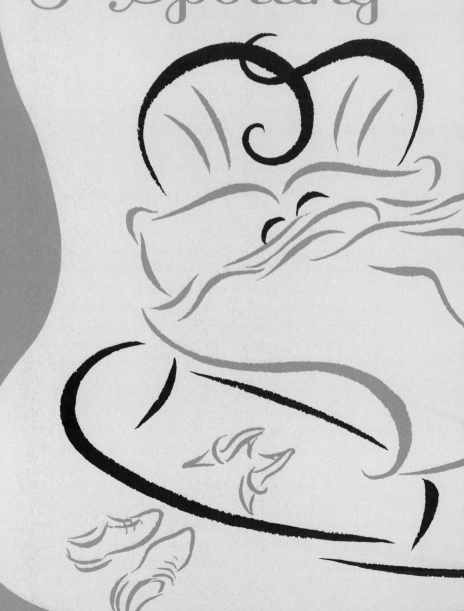

Even if you'd never found your G-spot, you must have at least heard of it before reading this book. The P-spot, on the other hand, is a new one for most women. What is the P-spot? How do you get there? Is it like the G-spot, only farther down the alphabet? First and foremost, understand this: no matter how far you delve into yourself—spiritually, intellectually, physically—you won't find it. It's not possible. But why, you ask? The P-spot is not located in you. It is found, exclusively, in men.

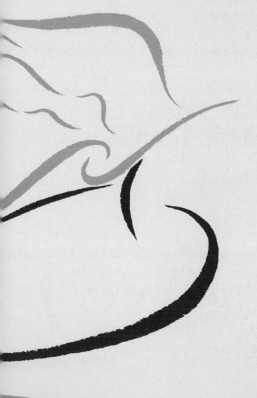

What Is It?

The "P" stands for prostate gland. In Salons, I've seen more than a few women look very tense, afraid, and nervous when I bring up the prostate, or P-spot. Maybe they think I'm rehashing the bit about the sensation of having to pee during intercourse ("pee," "P," the spoken word can be so confusing). Or maybe they'd only heard "prostate" connected with another word—"cancer." Hence the wincing. And then, as if the association with peeing and cancer isn't cringe-worthy enough, most women do have a vague sense that one accesses the prostate by putting a finger up a man's rectum, as if they'll need a proctology degree to find it. Barring that, they'd have to go exploring without credentials, a lab coat, protective headgear, or a sterile surgical environment.

What we do in the name of pleasure, I'm telling you.

The truth is, regardless of where it is, the prostate (otherwise known as the male G-spot) is an extremely sensitive heat-trigger for men, most of whom don't even know that their seminal fluid–producing gland is an explosive erogenous zone.

Gland to Meet You

Why is the prostate gland a well-kept secret of lust life? Of course, our culture is anally retentive. Americans are, as a people, very mum about the bum. The ass is the final frontier for sexual adventure and a no-man's land for casual conversation. Until age 10, fart and poop jokes are socially acceptable and for the most part, that's the extent of talk when it comes to the tush. The very idea of talking about the tush is unappealing isn't it? The thought of tush talk raises fears that something gross is about to be said.

Clearly the reticence we have about our nether regions includes the butt. In the next chapter of this book, I'll take on that subject in detail.

For now, suffice it to say that since the prostate is in the butt region, it is clouded in mystery, cloaked in the hush of tush.

Despite the under-the-radar PR on the P-spot, the prostate is a well-documented joy button throughout history. According to Stefan Bechtel et al., authors of *Sex: A Man's Guide*, World War II American military medics would give prostate massages to service men who hadn't been with women in months to release "pelvic congestion," an apparent euphemism for "unbearable horniness." At the turn of the century, women were urged to buy prostate massagers (small steel rods) to service their husbands during intercourse. Thanks to the dozens of books on Taoism and Tantra I've read, I can trace prostate play back to the ninth century.

Whoever said "There is nothing new under the sun," was right. But rediscovery can be the mother of invention. Just because men have always had prostates (just as women have always had clitorises), doesn't mean that we should stop searching for innovative ways to capitalize on their God-given pleasure production.

Prostate Overview

1. **The prostate is the key to male ejaculation.**

2. **The nerves that surround the prostate are essential for male erection.**

3. **Massage the prostate and even jaded men will be blown away.**

As you see in the illustration below, the prostate is a walnut-sized nugget of gland and muscle that is surrounded by nerves and erectile tissue. The bladder is right above it, and the pubococcygeus (PC) muscle floor is below; the prostate is behind the pubic bone (just a little further back than the G-spot is in women) and just in front of the rectum. It's at the center—the epicenter—of a man's internal sexual organs. Sperm travels from the testicles through the vas deferens tubes

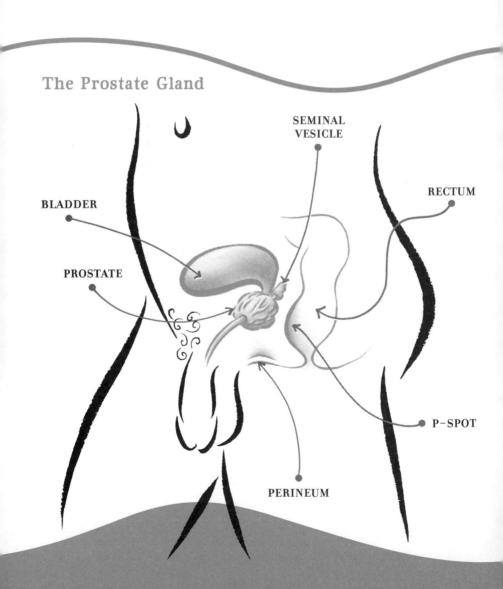

The Prostate Gland

SEMINAL VESICLE

RECTUM

BLADDER

PROSTATE

P-SPOT

PERINEUM

to the seminal vesicles, where 50 percent of the ejaculatory fluid is produced before moving through the prostate. A micro-factory, the prostate produces an enzyme-rich milky substance that completes the semen, and then, thanks to its muscle, contractions release the finished product. Otherwise known as ejaculation or, the technical phrase, spurting love juice.

Without the contribution of the prostate (the milky enzyme-laden fluid), the sperm from the testicles would be clueless about locating eggs. One prostate-producing enzyme, PSAP, helps the semen clot so that it can stay where it's deposited, deep in the vagina near the cervix. Once the clotted semen is in place, the other prostate-produced enzyme, PSA, kicks in to dissolve the surrounding fluid, setting the sperm free to plunder the cervix. In addition to these clotting and dissolving enzymes, the prostatic fluid contains essential minerals, including calcium and zinc (the jury is still out on their exact role).

The two nerves that surround the prostate are the last link in the chain reaction of messages from the brain to the spine to the erectile tissue in the penis that needs to "get hard" at the same time it needs blood to flow into the erectile tissue to make it happen. If anything happens to those nerves, brain to penis communication is in jeopardy as is the necessary blood flow for erection. The chance of harming those two essential nerves during prostate surgery is historically very high. Which is why, when oncologists talk about removing a cancerous prostate, men beg for other options. Actually, they needn't worry as much as in the past. A new surgical technique has been developed in the past ten years whereby surgeons can remove the cancerous organ and still preserve the nerves around it. While we're on the subject, prostate cancer stats are similar to those of breast cancer. According to the American Cancer Society, one in six men will develop prostate cancer in their lifetimes (one in eight women get breast cancer). Prostate cancer, like breast cancer, is not contagious. You can't catch cancer from a prostate, whether healthy or unhealthy. Touching it does not put your partner at increased risk of prostate cancer, just as his touching your breasts is not a carcinogenic activity. Okay? Okay.

Now that I've dispatched with those concerns, let's move along to other worries, like, how do you get to the prostate and those sensitive, fabulous nerves, and once you're there, what do you do?

The P/G Connection

The P-spot and the G-spot have a lot in common. I'll start at the beginnings, the very origins of humanity. Remember way back when you were an embryo? You don't? Well, while you were otherwise occupied, sucking down amniotic fluid and splitting cell nuclei, your reproductive organs were taking shape. All embryos start out female, with the same basic infrastructure, nerves, and tissue types. They all look exactly the same. Embryos with a Y chromosome then morph into the sex organs you can plainly see on the guy next to you in bed at night. It may sound like late night on the Sci-Fi channel, but it happens every day in pregnant women all over the world. The clitoris becomes the penis. The ovaries become the testicles.

Fetal Genitalia

UNDIFFERENTIATED EMBRYO BEFORE THE SEVENTH WEEK

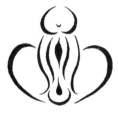

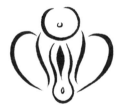

EMBRYONIC REPRODUCTIVE ORGANS EVOLVING INTO MALE OR FEMALE GENITALIA

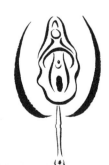

Even the uterus and vagina remain, albeit undeveloped, becoming the "prostatic utricle" also known as "uterus masculinus" or male uterus. It's is a small pouch of would-be uterus and vagina about a quarter of an inch long invisible to the eye because it's located in the center area of the prostate. The G-spot morphs into the prostate gland. But since the prostate has had more attention and produces a specific fluid, the G-spot is also known now as "the female prostate" because it turns out that the ejaculatory fluid of both sexes is the same. In fact, female "paraurethral glands" and ducts are 20–25 percent lighter but function the same as the ducts and glands that make up the prostate, producing the same fluid.

To stimulate the G-spot, as described in chapter 3, the owner needs to be aroused already (check back to page 55 for details). Same thing with the P-spot. But, unlike G-spotting, P-spot stimulation can be achieved externally. Get it? From outside the body. No penetrating of

Consider the similarities between the G-spot and the P-spot:

✳ **Both are the size of a walnut and are made up of textured erectile tissue that swells with arousal.**

✳ **Both are located between the bladder and the penis/clitoris.**

✳ **Both are wrapped around the urethra.**

✳ **Both produce ejaculatory fluid.**

✳ **Both are pleasure centers with nerves connecting to the clitoris/penis.**

✳ **Both respond to direct stimulation by producing intense orgasms.**

orifices necessary. Need I spell it out even more clearly? You can get at the prostate without having to insert a single fingernail into a man's ass. WHEW!! I'm sure you're feeling much better about the whole enterprise now.

The prostate, as mentioned above, is blanketed by highly sensitive nerves that are the basis of all male sexual pleasure. Get at those nerves with massage and it's like mainlining erotic heroin. Fortunately, the prostate rests directly on top of the perineum. Another p-word, the perineum is a band of flesh that runs from the base of the scrotal sac to the anus (in fact, this stretch of sensual highway is often called the "taint," as in, "it ain't the balls and it ain't the butt"). Women have one, too, running from the vulva to the anus. The perineum has plenty of nerve endings of its own for everyone, so rubbing the area on a man is a two-for-one deal, stimulating the perineal nerves directly and the prostate indirectly.

For an outside job: go straight to the perineum. Make circles with your fingers on that smooth area. Feel for a small indentation under the skin about three-quarters of the way down from the scrotum. The prostate is right above that dent.

Lubrication is always a handy helper, especially in this event. For one thing, men don't self-lubricate the way women do. And for another, in all sexual matters, friction is not your friend. Use lubrication made for sex though. Hand cream, Vaseline, and baby oil can lead to vaginal irritation or infection and/or degradation of a condom, which defeats the purpose. For a run-down of good lubrication options, go to page 121 in chapter 6.

After you've lubed up, start with the circular motion on the perineum (gently yet firmly). Press upward (slowly yet purposefully), and you can feel the prostate itself. But don't focus exclusively on the "prostate above" dimple mentioned here. The whole area is a hot patch for men, a red-hot one. Don't press too hard though. You're not massaging his strong, beefy shoulder muscles or his strapping manly legs. This is a delicate little gland and area and needs to be handled with care and respect. Combine external P-spotting with a hand job or blowjob and you'll make a friend for life.

For more direct, and therefore more intense, P-spotting, it takes an inside job. Those willing to go for a more direct route will have to venture into uncharted waters and penetrate their boyfriend's body, but not very much. The prostate is not, of course, inside the rectum. It is very near the rectal wall (just like the G-spot is on the other side of the vaginal wall), on the downward stomach side. You can feel it pretty easily two or three inches in (reachable with even the most lady-like index finger). The walnut shape is distinctive. Texturally, it's softer—more sponge than shell.

Nuts and bolts approach details: lube up (a lot) his anus and your finger. Have him lie on his back. Sit between his legs. Slowly insert finger. Very slowly. Palm up so you can hook your digit toward his stomach side. Experiment with gentle circles and up-down strokes. See what your partner likes. You can use a latex glove or not, but be sure to have cut nails and lots of lubricant. No lubricant equals no fun. I simply cannot stress enough the benefits of lubrication. Combine internal P-spotting with a blowjob or hand job and you'll have a slave for life.

That Is, If He's Willing

All well and good, you say. I'd love a man-slave for life, you say. But meanwhile you may be thinking, "My guy would never let me near his butt. No fucking way." A lot of women have said this to me at Salons. "I accidentally got near his butt once and he freaked out," one confessed.

There *are* a lot of scared guys out there. They don't always know what's good for them. Any sudden movements in that area can certainly make a guy freak out. Men tend to have three main barriers about any kind of tush activity:

1. FEAR OF PAIN
2. FEAR OF THE UNKNOWN
3. FEAR OF LIKING IT

Start with the *assumption* that you and he have nothing to fear but fear itself. All mental barriers can be dismantled with open and honest conversation. And I'm going to tell you exactly how to converse with him for his own benefit. He'll want to thank me later. He can send an e-mail to comments@safina.com.

BARRIER NUMBER 1: Fear of Pain

Many men have had only one previous prostate experience. That involved a doctor, rubber gloves, and a cold examining room. About as far from erotic as one can get. And since he wasn't getting any pleasure from the exam, he probably resisted the intrusion, and that might equal pain on insertion. Any woman who's had a decidedly unsexy, uncomfortable time getting a pap smear can relate. Just the word "speculum" can make a woman close up tighter than a fist.

Your mission, should you choose to accept it, is to drive home the point that you're not giving him a health check, the bed is not an examining room table, your womanly touch is not that of a hairy-handed doctor. You will be gentle and caring, not medical and mechanical. There will be no snapping of rubber gloves, only the soft panting of hot and heavy lovemaking. Go slooowwwly. And ask repeatedly in the hot and heavy spirit of the moment if he is okay as you progress.

BARRIER NUMBER 2: Fear of the Unknown

The fear of the unknown includes fear of pain, but mostly it's just not knowing what to expect. Your guy may believe that prostate massage is kinky, dirty, awkward, gross. His hesitation is similar to ordering a strange sounding dish at a restaurant; will he like it or be disgusted by it? He just doesn't know, and, frankly, neither do you. Of course, most of his reluctance is specifically ass related. Consider if you said to him, "Let me rub you in a new spot between your toes. I read in this awesome sex book that it will drive you crazy." How fast do you think his shoe would be off? Make the comparison to him. Remind him of the first time he tried sushi. The first time he snowboarded. Only the brave are rewarded in this world. That includes you too. Your intrepid sense of exploration may inspire him. Your enthusiasm (if it's genuine) will be contagious. Someone else's confidence and assurance may be all he (or you) needs to let fun override fear.

"If I like it, does that mean I'm gay?" You know that's what he's thinking. Any interest in his own ass, or even your ass, might convince an unworldly man that he has latent homosexual tendencies and that he'd rather not go anywhere near that bend of thinking. He will drop the subject summarily and refuse to discuss it. Examine the twisted logic in this double whammy of shame: he's afraid of liking something that might mean he's gay, but he's afraid to admit those fears because the notion alone might lessen him in your eyes. Would you want to "make him gay" by probing his prostate? No, but we're not talking about rational thinking.

It may sound ridiculous, but some men are very hung up on their masculinity. "Butt Touching + Liking It = Gay" is a deeply rooted equation for many American men. Even though very enlightened men know rationally that this is bullshit, some can't help where their minds take them.

Just to be sure everyone's on the same page here, touching yourself or being touched anywhere on your body does not affect which gender you prefer to be touched by. There aren't parts of your body that will make you more interested in sleeping with the same sex if they're stimulated. Lesbians give oral sex to other women. Are you a lesbian for liking it when he goes down on you? Gay men give blowjobs. Does that mean he's gay for liking it when you do it? Every part, zone, spot you've got should be enjoyed. Same for him. No one "goes gay" from his own happy nerve endings. Not that there would be anything wrong with that, but it doesn't happen by flicking a switch.

P-spotting for His Health

This last argument might convince him. According to the Prostatitis Foundation, prostate massage "has the effect of getting rid of built-up pus and dead cells, and shrinking the gland, relieving symptoms" of many inflamed prostates. This method was used pre-1960, before antibiotics were widely administered, and this method is still practiced with success. So not only can a P-spot tweak maintain a healthy prostate, it may cure an inflamed one too.

Communication

Convincing him to try something new brings up an even larger subject: how to communicate effectively with your partner about sex. As a blanket statement, reading this book will probably make you a lot more educated about your body, his body, sexual adventure, and response than he is. No one likes to be talked down to. So when you bring up things you've learned, be sure to blame me for everything. Show him pages from the book. Leave the book in the bathroom where he's sure to peek at it.

Also, as mentioned previously, be assured that men like it when you talk about sex. They like how it sounds; they like to imagine doing what you're discussing. Hearing you use key words is probably one of his fantasies (hint: those words are not "stop," "ouch," and "headache"). When you decide to launch a conversation about what you'd like to try and why, keep the tone enthusiastic, with the honest innocence of nasty fun.

You've probably heard not to bring up wild new tricks when you're already in bed. True, that might throw him off his stride, making him wonder if you hate what he's doing *right now.* Outside-the-bedroom talk, simply because it's not in the sex chamber, has an extra erotic flavor. I like to have these conversations in the kitchen over breakfast. Start the day with a healthy appetite and let it grow until nighttime when talk can turn into action. If breakfast is too much, do it while having dinner. Come to think of it, talking about sex while eating may be the sexiest combination of all, with moving mouths and savory tastes. Ah, yes. I may have to stop writing now and meet a man for dinner…

Where was I? Yes, the reciprocity of sex talk. It's wonderful to be able to talk about it. It's even more wonderful when you can listen too. You've got to be confident enough to listen to what he wants to say. This is the hardest part of communicating for most people. If you don't create an atmosphere of receptivity, your partner won't be able to reveal things to you for fear that you will judge or dismiss him. This is true when you have the third-date sexually transmitted disease discussion (which I sincerely hope you have/will have before sleeping with anyone), and it's true later on when you talk about fantasies, P-spotting, and beyond. Show your openness by shutting up when he talks and by nodding and smiling to encourage him. He should do the same for you. Don't interrupt him or wave off his concerns. Listen, smile, and nod, and then you'll get your turn. If you show him courtesy, he'll hand it back to you, and then some.

Minds Wide Open

Men and women—people I hardly know—tell me their most intimate secrets. They sense that I have an open mind and that I'm not going to reject them or judge them. If you let go of feeling threatened and focus on being interested in what your partner wants or thinks about (which I'm sure you are), he'll sense you have an open mind too. The more open the better. For sex, and love.

There were so many things I wanted to do with my wife but I just knew she wouldn't be interested, that she would think I was deviant and weird. Maybe I am. I know how scared I am. But that didn't change what I wanted to do with her. I got obsessed with my ideas and wanted to do them with anyone after awhile. Finally, after fourteen years of being married to her, I did do these things with someone else and it was such a relief. I realized that I can't be me in my marriage and we're getting a divorce.
—Mark, 42

Mark told me this last year. He also told me what his obsessions were. Honestly, a little light bondage just isn't that deviant. I'll bet dollars to doughnuts his wife would have gone along if they had worked out some rules beforehand. And their marriage would have been saved.

The blame lies with Mark's inability to communicate, but he must have been picking up judgmental signals from his wife too. What ended the marriage wasn't the lack of sex itself. It was the lack of communication. No telling if they would have come to a sexual impasse or not, since the conversation never happened. It may come to pass that, for all your encouragement, he suggests a sexual activity you do not want to do. Try to negotiate, find some wiggle room, compromise to meet everyone's needs. But if you can't come to an agreement and the relationship can't withstand your differences, at least you were both honest and considerate instead of distant and secretive. Isn't that a better, more mature way to go out than living in shame and fear? You bet it is, and you'll be that much more prepared to start a new relationship.

The Male Multiple Orgasm

Women can flow from one orgasm to the next because we don't require recovery time. The blood rushes to our genitals, muscles spasm, tension is released, blood flows away. But with breathing and focus, the blood can flow immediately back and women can come again.

Men have a different experience. Blood rushes to their genitals, muscles spasm, the penis ejaculates. With ejaculation, semen spurts and blood rushes out of the penis (all that blood is what makes it hard in the first place). He goes limp and needs a resting period to get hard again.

HOWEVER, it is possible—but not easy—for men to have the muscle spasm without ejaculation. Disconnecting the two reflexes, allowing muscle spasm but delaying ejaculation, is the basis of a male multiple orgasm (MMO). His multiple orgasm, to clarify, isn't repeated ejaculation. No man alive can spew his load and then twenty seconds later live to spew again. MMO is all about making orgasm and ejaculation two separate things. To prolong his pleasure by traversing a landscape of little peaks that eventually reach a heavenly summit, as opposed to the usual scaling Mount Everest then exploding and collapsing. Similar but different from women's multiple orgasms.

Separating muscle spasm from ejaculation is a very old idea actually. MMO was originally introduced in Chinese Taoist philosophy during the Chou Dynasty (770–222 B.C.). It's way too complicated to explain in detail, but suffice it to say, much of those teachings were incorporated into Tantra, an Eastern sexual practice made famous by Sting and his wife Trudy. Basically, the Taoists believed everyone has yin and yang energies inside them and that both forces must be in balance for a person to be healthy. Yang is male, yin is female. You've probably seen the Taoist black and white circle symbol, a white paisley with a black spot hugged against a black paisley with a white spot. To get more yin (female) energy, men were taught to have sex as often as possible but to hold off on ejaculating, which would let go of too much yang (the male energy that they thought they had limited supplies of). So men started practicing sex techniques that allowed them to absorb a lot of yin (from female orgasms) without ejaculating out their yang. In other words, they learned to separate their own orgasm spasms from ejaculation.

MMO dates back to a time when sexual fluids were considered "sacred" and part of religious ritual. Masturbation was considered a dangerous waste of male or female energy. Of course, nowadays we know that our fluids are forever self-replenishing and that masturbation keeps our organs in proper working order. Some of the attitudes from ancient times are best left in the past. But there are also bits of gold among the dross. MMO is a solid chunk of the good stuff.

Male Multiple Orgasm for NOW

MMO is counterintuitive. Why delay ejaculation when it feels so excellent? Imagine, if you will, delaying that pleasure, prolonging and stretching the tension, hanging on the edge of explosion (the best part), and then, after all that, having a volcanic meltdown that will make you believe wholeheartedly in the glory of God and true love? Yeah, why would anyone want to do *that*?

Granted, you don't get such joys easily. It takes study and commitment. For a man to learn to separate his orgasm spasms from ejaculation he has to practice on his own, just like you need to locate your G-spot for yourself before you can reliably show him. Once he's practiced a bit, here's what the two of you can try:

1. By intercourse or other methods, he should get to the point just before orgasm and stop, but not in the "quick, think about baseball" method he probably uses now. This is a physical cessation. As he starts to orgasm/spasm, he should clench his PC muscles. The PC muscles are what men and women use to stop the flow of urine. On men, tightened PC muscles can cut off the flow of ejaculatory fluid from the prostate.

2. You can't do anything about his PC muscle strength (Kegel exercises will do wonders for him too, but you should stop stimulating his penis while he's clenching his PC muscles by staying still. Drop whatever you're doing, and he'll have an easier time containing himself. He can tell you to hold off by giving you a signal (a word, a squeeze), or you can feel when it's time to hold off when you feel the base of the penis start to rumble. Developing a signal system is just another way to communicate well and improve intimacy, stay in the moment, and keep enjoying yourselves. Remember too that this is all in good fun. Nothing could be worse than approaching sex like a job that has to be done right. Stay in the spirit of things or the spell will be broken.

3. Position allowing, at that first rumble, firmly press upward on his prostate (yes, via the anus). This move is called "the finger lock" by Douglas and Rachel Abrams, authors of *The Multi-Orgasmic Man.* Use the three middle fingers of your right hand, press upward, and hold. Err on the side of gentleness, of course. It's much more important not to hurt him than to stop his prostate from releasing fluid. He can let you know if pressing harder would be okay next time. And there should be a next time. The fun is in the trying as much as the succeeding, as long as you and your partner agree to look at it that way.

Also keep in mind that prostate trouble can start or be worsened by fluid buildup within the gland. Regular ejaculation helps wash out those fluids, and researchers suggest that sudden changes in ejaculation frequency can trigger prostate problems. So keep all good things in moderation as usual.

A Top Ten List of Other, Less Trodden Erogenous Zones

1. His chin
2. The path between his earlobes and the hollow by his collarbone
3. The nape of his neck
4. The inside of his elbows
5. The length of his spine
6. His inner thighs
7. The pulse points on his wrists
8. The space between his fingers and toes
9. His balls—some men love to have them cradled or kissed
10. His hair—gently lifted away from the scalp and slowly released all over his head

Tush Talk

When I hit junior high school, I started to see boys as sexual objects. My girlfriends and I hashed over their attributes and spent hours arguing about which boy was the "cutest." We actually constructed a point system based on their hair, eyes, smiles (point detracted for braces), and clothes (we worked within the narrow

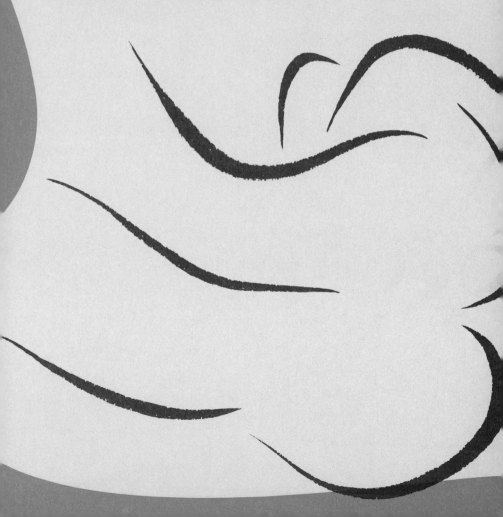

range of style for the Hampton Middle School). Should a boy successfully meet our minimal point requirements, we would then turn our conversation to deeper, more important masculine distinctions: his butt.

The ultimate compliment for a boy was, "He has a cute butt." The boys seemed to be aware that this appraisal carried extra weight. Of course, we didn't bother casting our eyes below a guy's belt if he had bad acne or dressed lamely. He had to qualify first on our ridiculous rating system. We never said, "He's a dog-faced loser, but what a great ass!" An attractive posterior was not a saving grace. It was the final vote of approval, the watershed element that turned an acceptable guy into a lust-worthy hottie.

Every woman can easily remember that one boy from eight grade—the one every girl in class found unattainably, intimidatingly desirable. And, I ask you now, looking back with the hindsight (as it were) of the years, whether that grade A boy had a grade A ass. Of course he did. He probably still does. Cue to sigh heavily like a 15-year-old girl.

Do NOT Go There

A man's ass. Indeed, it can be a beautiful thing. I openly admire men's rear ends on the subway, walking down the street, on line at Starbucks. But in terms of concrete (versus abstract) interest in a particular man, the cute butt issue is still an afterthought for me. He's got to be attractive in other areas first (surprisingly—shamefully?—many of those junior high qualifications still apply) before I survey his butt. Serious tush surveillance is, after all, deeply intimate. Considering the contours of his caboose is one small step away from thinking about touching it.

The butt is the hot seat of the American sex paradox. As a nation, we're fixated on it, constantly examining it (others and our own). We love high, round cheeks, not too flat and not too fat. A great behind can launch an international multimillion dollar entertainment industry (look at J.Lo). A sexy ass can be a national treasure (like Britney Spears's). We examine our own butts down to each dimple. We go to exercise classes that focus solely on the gluteus muscles (New York fitness guru Lottie Burke has made a singular career out of ass-lifting aerobics).

Despite the laser focus on the shape of our butts, we are mostly ignorant of the ass's inner workings. As a society, we maintain strict aversion to the butt's role in sex. We shy from probing it in depth. But(t), despite this, the subject of anal sex comes up, eventually, in every relationship. Usually, the man mentions it first. He may simply ask permission to go for it or start a discussion about it, as in, "Do you take it up the ass?" Or, more delicately put, "Have you ever, you know, done that, you know, the anal sex thing?" Shrieking in horror and humiliating him for asking (as in, "Of course not! What are you, some kind of latent homo pervert?") will *not* further your sexual or emotional intimacy. That said, you shouldn't just do it to please him. You should do it because you're curious or adventurous or looking for new ways to have fun in bed. Having the straight facts about anal sex/stimulation will be useful in any event. Ignorance is not always bliss. Sometimes ignorance is what stands in the way of bliss.

The Final Frontier

No one talks about anal sex. If your boyfriend/husband said he wanted to do it with you, would you call your friends to discuss the matter? From what I've heard at Safina Salons, this rarely happens. What's even rarer: women admitting that they enjoy anal sex, even if they do. They're ashamed of their interest in something they consider seedy or bizarre. Most women—of the women I've met, I'd say around 90 percent—find the idea of anal sex dangerous, dirty, and potentially painful.

When I began hosting Safina Salons and came face-to-face with such violent distaste for the subject, my first thought was to skirt the whole area as a topic of discussion. My second thought was to remind myself that the chief operating principle of my company is to get sex talk out in the open. Not to hold back. Not to make any sexual practice a taboo. Shying away from any pleasure source was antithetical to my ideals. I resolved to go there, to the butt. It was my job, my obligation, to explore the terrain most women feared to tread. How do people do it? How does it work anatomically? Emotionally? Hygienically? To get to the bottom of anal sex (as it were), I would have to open my own mind and then try to open the minds of others.

The Only Thing to Fear Is Fear Itself

Before I get into the nitty-gritty, I want to remind you all that you're just *reading* about anal sex here. Passing your eyes across words and sentences doesn't mean you've actually done anything sordid. Read with an intellectually hungry mind; consider the tantalizing possibility that there are pleasures you've never dared to exploit.

It's funny, even now, to talk blithely about pleasure in conjunction with such a place. After all, the anus is not a sexual organ per se. It's a digestive one. The phrases we associate with homosexual anal sex allude to this: "fudge packing," driving down the "Hershey highway." It's particularly unappealing when you put it that way, and the residue of hearing these things for years is in your head.

Now, if you must, please take a moment to giggle, grimace, and/or groan. Okay. Deep breath. Done? Good. Now say "ewww" and "gross" a few times. Excellent. Have you worked that out of your system? Have you put aside your primary, visceral reaction to anal sex? The next step: viewing the butt in a new bright, cheerful light so we can have a rational discussion about using it sexually without a negative cloud of distaste hanging over your mind.

As I mentioned above, I wavered on how to handle this subject in my early Safina Salons. Language, as always, is crucial. I decided to refer to the area as the "tush." This might seem a little silly. It is a little silly. How else to lighten the subject matter than by injecting a bit of silliness into the conversation? You can't say "tush" with dramatic weight. It's a light word, so I use it. "Butt" is a good alternative because it's neutral. While we are all very comfortable with the word "ass," it has a harsh edge to it. "Ass" still doubles as an insult. Certainly, "asshole" has the potency to offend. If I use "ass" at all, it's for effect. You can see how riled it makes you.

"Anal sex" and the equally unsavory "anus" give me the willies. It just sounds awful, clinical, medical, deviant. There's no measuring the nonsexy mood these words conjure. Plus, the ear isn't used to hearing them. I have rarely even heard anyone say "anal" or "anus" out loud. Who says such things, outside a proctologist or gynecologist's office? I've almost never heard them in conversation.

Henceforth, I'll use tush and butt mainly and try not to use the other words too often. That might help you get through this chapter in the proper frame of mind. After all, tush is fun. Butt has possibilities.

The Damage of Myths and Fear

As we grow up, girls learn next to nothing about the butt. Wipe front to back to avoid dreaded mysterious infections. Otherwise, zilch. Also, girls are quickly indoctrinated into the size issue (relating to the cheeks, not the opening): bigger is not better. The tush is dirty, bad, icky, and unsanitary. The negative messages from childhood stick. I had to force myself to seek out information on the subject because of my unquestioning acceptance of the tush taboo. I wasn't interested in knowing more because I thought I knew enough.

In truth, I knew nothing. I'd never had anal sex. I, myself, Shannon, the nice Midwesternish Irish-American girl, couldn't fathom the idea of doing *that*. Could having your butt penetrated feel good? I didn't think so, and I wasn't interested in finding out. The rectum seemed too small and dry for something as demanding as a penis. Maybe if I had a prostate, I thought (see chapter 5), then tush sex would have a point. But since I'm a woman, and therefore prostate-free, I didn't see what was in it for me. Besides which, as far as a man's interest went, why would he want to be a backdoor man when there was this lovely, well-lubricated vagina, front-and-center? I assumed that any woman who consented to have anal sex submitted to it for a man's pleasure alone, which was an even grosser thought than actually doing it.

But many women do like it. Some love it. And there are books to prove it. I found a couple that were dedicated exclusively to tush sex. The titles are off-putting. I didn't want to buy them in a bookstore (back to childhood embarrassment), so I ordered them online. They are *Anal Pleasure and Health: A Guide for Men and Women* by Jack Morin, M.D., and *The Ultimate Guide to Anal Sex for Women* by Tristan Taorimino. I found both very illuminating and worth reading.

The main benefit of my research was to normalize the idea of anal sex. This wasn't a perversion or aberration. Not to Dr. Morin and Taorimino, who is the queen of anal sex (and has made a cottage industry of it, selling same-themed videos starring porn actors as well as her book). Taorimino just loves it. She can't live without it. She says it's safe, painless, easy, nothing to be afraid of. Like anything unfamiliar, it's frightening until you try it. And then, once it's familiar, anal sex is downright normal.

Turns out, she's right. In the name of research, proving my dedication to Safina, I went out and got me some. I followed Taorimino's directions to a tee—lots of communication, lots of lubricant, and very slowly . . . So now that I've been indoctrinated, I'm able to put the myths and fears about tush sex aside. For your sake, I'll break them down and tackle them, one by one.

MYTH NO. 1: Tush Sex Is for Gay Men

It's not even necessarily for them. You'll probably be surprised to know that some of my gay male friends report that tush sex isn't part of all gay men's lives. What do they do instead? Blowjobs, hand jobs. In a recent study of how gay men self-identify regarding the activity, 18 percent didn't see themselves in any anal sex role (top, bottom, or versatile). The fact that there are gay men out there who don't want anyone near their butts makes plenty of sense when I think of it. After all, gay men grow up with the same negative messages we all got. Gay sex means carnal activity between two people of the same gender. Which sexual activity is besides the point, and not orientation-specific.

MYTH NO. 2: Tush Sex Is Perverted and Dirty

Once upon a time, not too long ago, a blowjob was an unspeakable act of perversion. In 1948, Alfred Kinsey found that fewer than half of the men he interviewed had any experience with fellatio or cunnilingus, even if they were married. John Updike published *Rabbit, Run*, his groundbreaking novel about infidelity, in 1960. The book climaxed with what was then a scandalous blowjob scene, portraying the act as the ultimate unobtainable desire of American men—and something a good wife would never do. The sexual liberation of the 1960s and the interest women started taking in having their own orgasms helped the cause of oral sex. By 1977, *Redbook* magazine reported that 93 percent of wives in their survey had received cunnilingus and 91 percent had performed fellatio. Following on the heels of the '70s, fear of HIV in the 1980s capped the transition of oral sex from slutty to acceptable to typical.

For the religious right and pregnancy-fearing teenagers, oral sex is a satisfying alternative to vaginal intercourse. These teens, in fact, don't count oral sex as "sex." Sex is still defined as vaginal intercourse by our culture. To wit, a 1991 Kinsey Institute study found that 60 percent of college students would not say they "had sex" if their activities were limited to mouth on genital; a 2002 survey by the makers of LifeStyles condoms reported that one-third of teenage girls said oral sex is not sex. Despite their not having "sex," teens are awful busy having "not sex." Twenty percent of them have oral sex by 15; half of all teens do it by 17.

The point to this blowjob digression? If fellatio was once a forbidden act, isn't it entirely possible that, a few years from now, tush sex will also transition from freaky to commonplace? The mainstreaming has already begun. In the first *Bridget Jones* movie, Renee Zellweger and Hugh Grant have a brief anal interlude. The 2003 movie *Bad Santa* had a running butt sex joke. Any straight porn movie made nowadays has as much anal action as vaginal. And according to reports from health care workers, more teens are having anal sex as an alternative to "real" sex to avoid pregnancy—and to maintain virginity. As more and more people do it, and talk about it (this may take a while), the word will get out on how to have tush sex safely and joyfully.

So much for the concept of perversion. As for tush sex's alleged "dirtiness," it is not much dirtier or germier than vaginal sex. Yes, there are bacteria in the butt. Yes, you need to be careful not to transfer anything between the vagina and anus, in either direction, or you may suffer, among other things, a urinary tract infection (which, as we all know, is painful as hell and to be avoided at all costs). You might not realize that the rectum is relatively clean. It's not a storage area for feces. Waste passes through it but isn't stored inside it. So unless you feel the urge to defecate, the rectum is devoid of matter. The rectum itself is about a foot long. Unless your partner's penis is more than twelve inches long, he won't come into contact with waste. To avoid the *fear* of dirt, take a shower or a bath. Use a baby wipe on yourself. And, as always, have your partner wear a latex condom. This eliminates worry and prevents the transmission of fluids. HIV is estimated to be ten times more easily transmitted to the receiver of tush sex than the giver. Condoms are not foolproof. Herpes and other sexually transmitted diseases are still transmittable even when he wears one. It's advisable for both partners to get tested for every possible disease first and to stay monogamous.

So butt sex is not perverse. It's not dirty. But what of the strangeness, the illogicalness? Anal sex is going in the out door. It's entering an exit. It just doesn't make sense, does it?

MYTH NO. 3: *Tush Sex Doesn't Make Sense*

When you think about it, the vagina is a two-way street. Penis in; baby out. But let's not limit sex to the reproductive. Sex is about sensation. There is not a person on this earth who hasn't felt powerfully wonderful tingling sensations at some point when—forgive my bluntness—she's taken a shit. This goes beyond psychological and intestinal satisfaction. The anus, you see, is densely packed with nerve endings.

Flash back to chapter 4. Recall the "excitement" phase of orgasm. Blood rushes to the genital region and causes vasocongestion, which leads to the erection of the penis, the engorgement of the clitoris, and the lubrication of the vagina. The anus, next-door neighbor to the vagina, two doors down from the clitoris, also goes through changes as you heat up. According to *Anal Pleasure and Health*'s Dr. Morin, during the excitement phase, the anal tissues also get a blood infusion and secrete moisture; the anal muscles spontaneously contract, and the nerve endings around the anus and along the perineum perk up.

It's all connected. The tush entrance is part of the pubococcygeus (PC) muscle floor. There are two anal sphincter muscles, one internal and one external. Both tighten and loosen, but one is voluntary and the other is involuntary. When in the excitement phase, just a wee bit of external stimulation (touching the anus manually) causes the anal muscles to expand involuntarily. Put pressure on the anus and it opens up. The tight pucker widens, nerve endings surge and tingle.

The tush gets just as happy and ready for sex as the vagina. It's crying out for attention. This is anatomical fact. Surprised? I was too.

We covered the prostate in chapter 5, so you can see the logic in tush excitement in men. For women, the evolutionary explanation for our anal sexual response is more mysterious. Regardless of the mystery, the facts are that the anus has a full load of nerve endings and that it pumps intensely during orgasm. If you haven't noticed that your anus does a wild dance when you come, it's probably because you haven't been paying attention. Most women don't. Resistance against the contractions (having something inside the anus) intensifies sensation. A finger will do. Once you've come with a finger in your tush, you may not want to go without again.

On www.puckerup.com, Tristan Taorimino's Web site devoted to anal sex, a woman expresses her fear that she isn't normal because, after fifteen years of marriage, she and her husband tried anal sex and now she prefers it to vaginal. Taorinimo welcomed her to the club and calmed her fears, writing, "The truth is that we like what we like." Amen to that.

MYTH NO. 4: Tush Sex Will Be Painful and Could Damage Me

It is, after all, a very tight hole. Insertion could hurt. Badly.

Not so. Consider the girth of fiber-formed stool. That's wider than a finger, and it doesn't hurt when it comes out. The butt is stretchy, just like the vagina. The vagina can enlarge enough to accommodate a ten-pound, twenty-inch long baby. The average penis is a mere six inches, with a diameter of a little more than two inches (the average circumference is almost five inches—which sounds like a lot until you think of how circumference is measured). In any case, the butt can handle it.

There is another fear regarding anal sex, but it doesn't get talked about much. What if doing it stretches the butt muscles permanently? Would that mean you'll have to start wearing adult diapers? Or if you do it too much, would you start walking with a limp? Or will your waste elimination process be impaired?

When done properly (e.g., slowly, lots of lubrication), tush penetration is 100 percent pain-free. There are no negative after effects. The anus is resilient and pliable and will return to its normal shape no matter what you do to it. Go slowly and use lubricant to prevent tearing the delicate skin. According to Taorimino, anal sex actually tones the sphincter muscles just as exercise tones any muscle group.

I think most of the fear of pain and damage comes from our connecting anal sex and sexual abuse: prison rape, pedophilia, and so on. When anal sex is forced upon someone, of course, it'll hurt and cause damage. This is also true of vaginal rape. Rape is not sex. It's a violent crime. If the only association you have of anal sex is rape, then it's no wonder the idea of doing it yourself is horrifying.

I did some research into our collective-unconscious fears of anal sex and quickly found the infamous eighteenth-century French author whose very name means pain and punishment. The Marquis de Sade (where the word "sadism"—getting sexual pleasure by inflicting pain on others—comes from) wrote many lengthy books and plays about sexual torture. De Sade was a big fan of extremely violent anal sex. His writings have filtered down through the centuries— whether you've read his stuff or not—inextricably linking pain with anal sex in popular culture. This link was easily reinforced by religious and legal laws that made anal sex between consenting adults, even married ones, a crime called sodomy. Incidentally, all oral sex is still a crime under the sodomy laws in Utah and Virginia and fourteen states have kept sodomy laws on their books despite a huge repeal movement around the country in 1980. The Supreme Court finally ruled sodomy laws unconstitutional on June 26, 2003.

Practicing and loving consensual sex of any kind shouldn't be a crime. Anal sex in particular isn't dirty, perverted, or illogical. It's an unexplored avenue to sensation. With patience, bravery, and lots of lubrication, a whole new world of pleasure can become available to you. I don't expect anyone to get in bed tonight and say to her partner, "Let's take the road not taken, sweetie." Sit on it for a while. Start slow with gentle touching. See where that takes you.

I used to gag at the idea of anal sex. The idea of a big hard-on ramming into that tiny tight hole—forget it. You're probably thinking I'm going to say "and then, one night ..." and it's probably cliché, but that's exactly how it happened. One night, my current boyfriend put his finger in my ass just a little when he was going down on me. My muscles gripped his finger, and it felt great. I came instantly. That was a hell of a shock. The next night, I asked him to do it again. And then he asked me about anal sex. I told him I was afraid. He assured me he'd be careful. First, he got me going with his fingers and some lube and then we did it. I have to admit, my anxiety made it tough for him to get in at first. I closed up as tight as a fist. So we did other things until I relaxed. When he finally got in, it felt great, to tell the truth. I was so surprised. Now, we use butt plugs and anal beads during vaginal sex. The anal stimulation combined with vaginal and clitoral is exquisite. What excites me the most about the anal play is that it still has a dangerous thrill to it. No matter how many times we do it, I still think of it as pushing the limits of normal. —*Stacy, 24*

Ten Truths about the Tush

1. The tush is involved in every orgasm whether or not you directly touch it.

2. Tush sex makes for intimate connections. You must agree to proceed and talk about what you're feeling while you're doing it.

3. The receiver has to be the one commanding the action.

4. Preparatory foreplay is needed, just like vaginal intercourse, but more so. The anal sphincter muscles will open, but they require stimulation first. Take your time. Never push or force.

5. The sphincters are muscles. Any exercise tones muscles. Anal sex is exercise for those muscles. It won't weaken them; it strengthens them.

6. A cultural taboo isn't correct merely because it exists. Women in the workforce were once considered "unnatural." Blowjobs were once the work of whores. Question your beliefs before you dismiss the practice outright.

7. One must wash (or change condoms) before switching finger or penis or sex toy from vagina to tush or the reverse.

8. The rectum is not a holding area for feces, and it's relatively clean. If you're in good health, have a thorough shower, and know that you don't need to have a bowel movement; there is no reason to have fears of messiness.

9. Using lubricant is required for comfortable tush sex. You can't be too thin, too rich, or have too much lubricant.

10. You don't need another person to explore your tush. Have adventures with your fingers or toys to improve your orgasms.

Step-by-Step Guide to Tush Play

1. **Use a lot of lubricant.**

2. **With a well-manicured, well-lubricated finger, rest it gently on and/or massage the anus while you do other things (e.g., oral sex, hand job, etc.).** The tush will open up on its own when it's ready. Use a latex glove to ensure cleanliness and to relax your mind.

3. **Never push your finger or anything else into someone's tush, and never let anyone push you.** Go slowly, and slide.

4. **Don't have tush sex if you're drunk.** Pain thresholds rise if you're blitzed or high, and you might wake up with a real pain in the ass.

5. **Never let go of anything you put near the tush.** This is a rule I can't believe is necessary to make, but I've heard too many stories of late-night trips to the emergency room. Once the tush gets excited, it starts sucking things in. Unlike the vagina, the colon is not a cul-de-sac. It's amazing but true that you have to keep a good hold on anything that goes inside the anus or you might find yourself saying to a triage nurse, "I put this vibrating egg in my boyfriend's butt, and all of a sudden, it was gone."

6. **Have fun.** Let the illicit associations power your passion, not squash it.

Lube Review

We have a little mantra at Safina, "More lube, better sex." If you don't already subscribe to this thinking, you won't be sorry if you adopt it. Lubricant makes sex smoother all around.

Two warnings: (1) household products not intended for sex—Vaseline, hand moisturizer, baby oil, butter—shouldn't be used. Some can degrade condoms and toys and/or they just shouldn't be inside you. Why risk a yeast infection or any other problem? Use real lubricant for safe fun; (2) lubricated condoms don't have enough lubricant for tush sex. You need to use more. Nonoxynol-9 was originally developed as a detergent and has been found to inhibit HIV, but it can irritate some people. If you find this is true for you, there are plenty of condoms out there without Nonoxynol-9, and no matter what, use more lubricant.

There are two main types of sex-safe lubricant: water-based and silicone. After looking at all the lubes out there, we decided that Safina should carry one water-based lubricant and one silicone-based lubricant for simplicity. Be assured that I picked the best. The water-based lubricant we sell is Liquid Silk; the silicone is Eros Bodyglide.

Water-Based Lubricants

✳ **Water-based means that the lubricant is less likely to cause yeast infections (one allergy warning: some contain glycerin—but not Liquid Silk).**

✳ **You can use it with any sex toys.**

✳ **Great for vaginal sex but less fabulous for tush sex. It tends to absorb into the skin and you need to keep adding more.**

We chose Liquid Silk because, as the promotional material reads, it "reduces friction in relationships." It's packaged like hand cream in an attractive pump bottle, and it really does feel like liquid silk. Val, my co-author, can't recommend it highly enough. She says it has changed her sex life.

Other popular water-based lubricants: Maximus, thicker than Liquid Silk; Astroglide; Wet; Eros Water Formulation; ID; O'My, which has hemp in it; Hydrasmooth comes in a hand cream—like tube; and Slippery Stuff. Many of these are available in flavors, which are fun, but don't use them if you're prone to yeast infections. The flavor comes from sugar, and that can set off a raging infection.

Silicone-Based Lubricants

✳ **Very concentrated. A little bit goes a long way.**

✳ **Thicker and more slippery feeling than water-based lubricants.**

✳ **Not to be used on silicone toys; it will degrade them.**

✳ **Great for anal sex because it stays slippery and won't absorb into the skin.**

I'm of the mind that water-based lubricant is best for vaginal sex and silicone-based lubricant is best for tush sex. I prefer Eros Bodyglide. Just a personal preference. Others include Wet Platinum, Bodyfluid, and Venus (also made by Eros).

Toy Stories

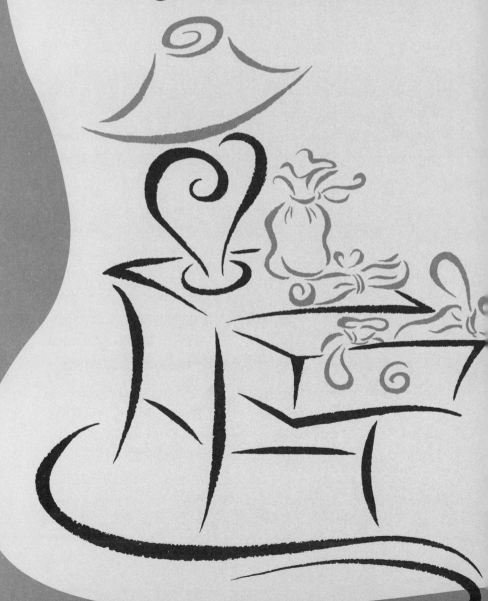

Chapter 7

Who's Afraid of Vibrator Shopping?

The words "sex toy" are off-putting to me. I immediately think of sleaze, deviance, and tastelessness. I may be a prude. Then again, sleaze may be what most Americans think when they hear "sex toy." I didn't feel comfortable with vibrators etcetera until recently. When I started Safina, which is fundamentally a sex toy business (although it is so much more), I owned only one very old and malfunctioning vibrator. My collection has since expanded.

Luckily, not everyone is as prudish as I am. I got my first glimpse at just how comfortable some of my contemporaries are on a sunny Saturday in June, about seven years ago. I'd just finished having brunch with a large group of friends, all in their mid-20s, my age at the time. As we shuffled out of the restaurant, Laura and I fell into step as we headed for the subway. I said I was going home. She announced that she was going vibrator shopping.

"What??" I sputtered. She was so matter-of-fact about it. It made me doubt I'd heard her correctly. My mouth fell open as she repeated herself.

"You're going to do that right now?" I asked in astonishment. Somehow, the idea of vibrator shopping in broad daylight seemed daring, risky, and aberrant.

"No time like the present!" she announced.

"How do you even know where to go?" I wondered out loud, starting to feel embarrassed for myself for being so provincial.

Instead of answering me, she urged me to tag along. We came to a corner storefront in Greenwich Village with lots of paraphernalia in the window. Laura walked up to the man at the cash register and asked smoothly to handle a few items in the locked glass case behind him. I peppered her with questions. How do you know what you're looking for? Which one works best? It costs how much? I must have sounded like a clueless child. She answered my questions matter-of-factly, as if we were handling kitchenware and not sexual appliances.

Despite Laura's ease, I was uncomfortable in that store. The room was bright, true. The sun filtered in, casting light, leaving no dark creepy corners. The men who worked there were nicely dressed gay men. The other customers were people who seemed just like Laura and me. But I was a prude, as I mentioned. I couldn't get over the wall-to-wall shrink-wrapped dismembered plastic penises. Vibrators were arranged in square plastic packs. Each one was endorsed with photos of the face (and other parts) of some porn star. These XXX women bulged out of their "clothes." The grotesque balloon breasts disgusted me. From between waxy lips, they stuck out their tongues, as if ready to lick the vibrator they held in their red talon fingernailed hands. "Yuck" was the first and only thought I had about this packaging.

After ten minutes of browsing and trying to cool down an embarrassed blush, I started to numb. The shock effect was wearing off, and I stopped feeling nervous and awkward. The chocolate penis lollipops looked jerky and stupid instead of threatening, and I felt jerky and stupid being there. These items and the packaging were desperately trying to be funny and sexy, but all I got was tacky, scary, or sad.

Laura, meanwhile, was shopping in earnest. She didn't seem to care about the pathetic attempt at humor and/or the depravity of the packaging as she searched for her next vibrator. She eventually chose an expensive Japanese vibrator that looked space age. It was smooth, white, not phallic-shaped at all, six inches long, a two inch wide tube capped in a flared red ball about three inches wide. A smooth, sleek tube, like one of the flares the ground control crews wave to guide planes to their gates. She was very pleased with it. I couldn't imagine how it worked or why she liked it so much. We left (finally), and Laura said she was going home right now to try it out.

"Right now??" I asked, shocked again. It was still a beautiful summer day. I was going to Central Park with a book. She smiled and rushed off, and I started wondering what I was missing.

One of the great flaws of this business is that thousands of sex toys designed for women are sold in stores that most women wouldn't dare walk into. Laura is exceptional. She has the balls, as it were, to walk in, suppress or ignore shame and shadiness, brave the bad part of town where these stores are often located, squint in the glaring theft-preventing lights, and gloss over the junky, ugly products and intimidating store staffers. Even the fat, lecherous-looking XXX store guys behind the counter reading porn magazines in typical sex toy stores don't ruffle her. She is on a mission, and nothing stops her. Few women have as much confidence.

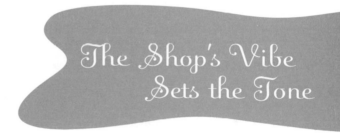

The Shop's Vibe Sets the Tone

Flash forward three years. While living in Belgium working for an international ad agency, I spent many weekends exploring Europe. I went to France, Germany, Italy. Amsterdam was a two-hour train ride away, and I relished its museums and street life.

On one such weekend, I was still in the center of Amsterdam's business district, but off the main streets, and I happened by a small store called Female and Partners. I couldn't tell what it was from the outside, so I stuck my head in. A tall, attractive woman with a big smile said, "Come in! Welcome!" She was smiling big at me. I had to go in or be a rude, ugly American.

There was skimpy red and black underwear hanging behind her so I thought it might be a kind of Frederick's of Hollywood lingerie boutique, but then I looked around. Vibrators were everywhere. But there were no male customers or XXX women on the packaging. Maybe this is a lesbian store, I thought. The woman sensed how awkward I felt and took it upon herself to put me at ease. She showed me a few things. She was very friendly and normal. The vibrators and other things were all sitting out on tables. I tolerated her commentary as I walked around the small space, trying to be polite and sincerely wondering what all the products were and how they differed from each other. Then she said, "Why don't you take a look at this wall. Let me know if you have any questions."

She was giving me my space, and I appreciated it. I examined the shelves, stared at the mysterious objects, some phallic and some mere lumps of plastic that reminded me of children's play-dough sculptures. I smiled at myself thinking how much Laura would like this place.

Then I saw a really attractive blue thing, six inches of blueness with trapped air bubbles inside that gave it dimension. It was a large oval shape that tapered off into two ripples that then curved into a rounded point about two inches wide. It wasn't crass or weird. It was beautiful; it was art. I wanted to touch it and see what it was made out of. "That one won a design award this year," the tall woman chimed from across the store. "It was made by a woman."

"Really?" I asked, amazed that there were design awards for vibrators and very pleased to know there was a woman making them. That information was all I needed to get to a point where I could actually purchase it.

"You have good taste," she said, as she wrapped my new award winning blue thing. "Expensive taste."

Specifically, $175.00 taste. But I didn't hesitate. If I were to buy a vibrator, any vibrator, it would have to be beautiful, an award winner, made by a woman, in cool, nonoffensive, space-age packaging. I felt like I'd joined the new century that hadn't quite started yet, like I'd caught up to my era as an independent, modern woman. I was now a vibrator owner! And there wasn't anything silly or stupid, sad or depraved about this blue thing.

I needed batteries, but quick. While guessing where I might get some in Amsterdam, I suddenly understood Laura's "right now" excitement about buying that Japanese vibrator all those years ago. I shared her excitement, but not her taste. I needed a sophisticated, cool store environment. I needed to be in a place that was tasteful so that I could relax and consider the products. The packaging also mattered to me, and a beautiful design was the clincher. This blue thing had form *and* function. This was a shopping experience I've always looked back fondly on.

I've based the shopping concept at Safina on that Amsterdam experience. Vibrator shopping shouldn't be any different than shoe shopping. A great shoe purchase will make you remember the experience of buying them. The store, the cute sales guy, the bargain you lucked into. A positive—nay, triumphant—shopping adventure can bring a smile to your lips weeks or years later. The memory of vibrator shopping at Female and Partners still makes me smile, and not just because a series of unforeseeable events on that one shopping day changed the course of my professional life.

A good vibrator shopping experience can change your life too, albeit in a less dramatic way. Take a minute now and separate your impressions of sex toy stores and bad packaging from the products themselves. Remove the sleaze from the stuff.

It's not a sex toy.
It's an accessory
for your lust life.

I don't sell "sex toys." I sell "Safina Sexories." I prefer thinking of vibrators etcetera as "accessories for your lust life." Referring to products that way is more cheerful. It's fun. Sex toys—as I call the large category of products—should be thought of as cheerful and fun. They are, after all. And how!

As you can tell from my story, I understand how awkward it can be to be curious and interested in learning more. And we all need to learn more, despite the awkwardness. That first vibrator opened my eyes to just how deeply women need sexual pleasure and guaranteed satisfaction for an overall healthy happy life. I quit my advertising agency job and set out to restructure the sex toy market on the model of a market like cosmetics because I realized that women need orgasms more than they need makeup, skincare, and hair care. They need orgasms as much as they need exercise, healthy food, and plenty of rest. Sexual pleasure and satisfaction relieve stress and increase health. I've beaten this drum since chapter 1, as you know.

The salubriousness of sex toys, however, is only half of the Safina mission. Getting over the sleaze factor is the other half. Products have to be the best, most attractive ones out there, and they have to be presented in a high-end, aspirational fashion that delights the eyes, lifts one's mood, and is luxurious and practical. With these ideas in mind, every Safina product comes wrapped in a shimmering, silky, custom-made, blue and silver bag. When you open your night table drawer, you'll see these shiny blue bags sitting cheerfully like presents in a row (NEVER will a Safina Sexory arrive in sleazy, embarrassing porn star packaging). The bags are an inducement to reach inside them again and again. At least, that's how it works for me.

An Overview of Sex Toys

There are thousands of products out there. It's overwhelming to walk into any sex toy store and see such a selection. The task of selecting the best, most attractive, and functional products for Safina to sell was daunting indeed. To manage the job, I broke down the products we sell (not *only* toys) into the categories of vibrators, tush toys, tie me up/tie me down, lotions and potions, games, and books and videos.

GOOD VIBRATORS—FABULOUS FEELINGS

Vibration—anywhere on the body—feels exciting and relaxing at the same time. A shiatsu chair in Sharper Image works the same way as a battery-sized handheld vibrator, or vibe. They both vibrate, but only one relieves stress down to the core of your being, makes you come, is affordable, and doesn't take up half your living room space.

Two things:

You don't want to vibrate a blood clot. That would be bad. See a doctor for pain. See a vibrator for pleasure.

You will not be "ruined" for fingers or dick or anything else if you use a vibrator. Repeat after me, once more, with feeling: vibrators excite nerve endings, they do not dull them.

At Safina, we sell several types of vibes: general "fun vibes" are for clitoral stimulation. They can be dildo shaped or made to look like lipstick. Some are plug-in wands—the kind of "massager" one can buy at Brookstone, say, or Sharper Image. There are vibrators that fit in your underwear and that are controlled by a remote held by someone up to twelve feet away. And there are small dolphin-, rabbit-, and bear-shaped vibes to put a smile on your face. There are vibrating fingertip covers and vibes that fit in the palm of your hand. The universe of vibrators is vast and ever-expanding. Why not, when they provide cosmic type experiences? Dual vibes are designed specifically to stimulate the clitoris and the G-spot/vagina at the same time. You could use this type of vibe on its own or while engaging in tush activity. Speaking of the back door, you can use a dual vibe in/around the tush and perineum, but just be sure that you decide where you're going to use it and stick to that decision. Sex toys are similar to the concept of keeping kosher. You have the tush toys and the vaginal toys, and a vibe that goes in the tush should never go in the vagina and vice versa. You can use condoms to prevent bacterial transfers (need I mention the threat of infection again?) and for easy cleanup, but it's best to keep your sex toys kosher. Why risk ruining the fun?

G-spot vibes are curved to better access the G-spot. You can use an additional small vibrator on the clitoris at the same time, or you can use your free hand or your partner's free hand. Waterproof vibes can be taken into the shower or bathtub. They also do well on dry land. The selection is limited, but you can find a range of colors and sizes. We sell a waterproof glove with little vibrators built into the pads of the fingers. It's great to use as a neck massager, but it can be used anywhere on the body in or out of the tub.

WHEN TO USE A VIBE **Seems to me, you can whip out a vibe nearly anywhere you have privacy.**
Usually though, they're excellent when you're stressed, randy, or bored. Or dirty. Or in bed with your partner.

When you're dirty. Why not keep a waterproof vibe in the shower? Every morning, you can give yourself a natural mood lift that will make your aromatherapy shampoo pale in comparison. A waterproof vibe is also a lot easier (and safer) than slippery shower sex.

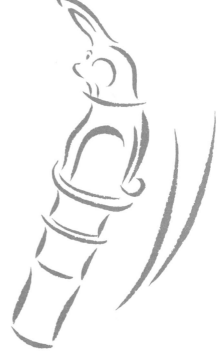

When you feel stressed, bored, or a little down. A little vibrating massage can take the tension out of your head, clear your sinuses, and make unimportant hassles look like minor chores. As you know by now, orgasms give you a positive outlook and a more balanced perspective.

When you need an easy-as-pie orgasm. Your partner may be fantastic, but your sexual gratification should not depend solely on him. This puts too much of a burden on the relationship, besides which, he may not be around when you really need an orgasm. There are vibrators so strong that you don't even have to take your clothes off to have a great time. You can come home from a bad day at work with the dreaded grocery shopping still ahead. Before going out to the market, press the Sure Thing vibe against your jeans for a few minutes, and you'll be the happiest, most energetic shopper in produce.

When you're in bed. I love to have a man on one side of the bed and a vibrator on the other. Why should we have to depend on him alone for me to come? And let's be honest, there are times in every girl's life when only a vibrator can get the job done. He can get in on the action too, with a hands-free vibrator. We sell one that's a jelly ring with a little vibrator on top. The ring fits around the base of his penis, and during intercourse, every deep thrust is a big buzz for you. This vibrator takes bumping and grinding to a whole new level. You can also hold a small vibrator to the clitoris during intercourse. We sell a few that will fit perfectly between two bodies in congress. As I've said before, less than 30 percent of women have orgasms during intercourse. While it's very good to be sure that you have orgasms before and after intercourse, since there's no orgasm limit, why not have some during intercourse too? Add a little vibration and have an even better time.

"HE'LL NEVER GO FOR IT" **I can't tell you how many times women have said this of their partners.**

They think men fear vibrators. A vibrator is an accessory. It's like a spice. You can have a great dinner with just salt and pepper, but a little spice can really add to your enjoyment of the main dish. Vibrators are simply part of the variety and fun of giving and receiving pleasure. It's important to talk to your partner about this and to let him know how you see vibrators fitting into your sex life. Some guys haven't thought through the idea. As usual, the unknown creates fear, and men are often afraid of bringing vibrators into you're their sex life. Here are some of men's fears about it. They might not admit to having some of them (not wanting to sound insecure or needy), but chances are, nearly every man has at least one of the following anxieties.

"THE VIBRATOR DOES THINGS I CAN'T DO. HOW CAN I COMPETE?" You know that the feeling of a vibrator is nice, but it doesn't compare to the feeling of a living, breathing person you care about.

You don't have chemistry with a machine. You'll never want to hug it and cuddle up to it or get up and cook it breakfast. It may help an orgasm along, but it won't make you feel any of the powerful emotions your lover evokes. Having an orgasm with the help of a vibrator is not about comparison or competiion. Make sure he knows this is how you feel.

"WHAT IF THE VIBRATOR DESENSITIZES YOU?" This fear is based on a misunderstanding of how nerve endings work.

Nerve endings don't get accustomed to anything but continuous stimulation (so if you held a vibrator to your clitoris without moving for a long time then, yes, it would get a bit numb). Once you stop stimulation, the nerve endings bounce back after a minute's rest as if they'd never felt a thing. I've been stubbing my toe on this step in my living room for years. And every time I do it, it hurts like the first time. The clitoris is no different than my toe. Nothing to worry about.

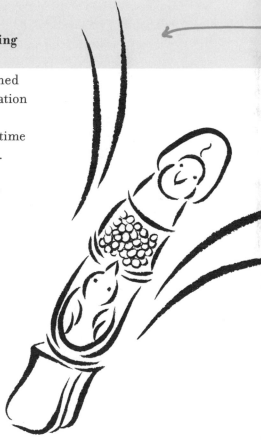

"BUT I WANT TO MAKE YOU COME ON MY OWN . . . "
An orgasm is an orgasm is an orgasm.

A vibrator just gives a man more options. He is involved, even in a vibrator orgasm. The vibrator doesn't find the right spot on its own. Someone is controlling it. Also, as we know, most women don't orgasm through intercourse alone. Why let frustration into the act when there are ways to ensure everyone's happiness?

"YOU DON'T NEED ME; YOU COULD JUST DO IT ON YOUR OWN . . . " **A first cousin to the paragraph above.**

When you have an itch and you scratch your own back, it feels nice, right? But it doesn't compare to when someone else does it—whether they use their hand or a back scratcher. Nerve endings doing their thing again. When you touch yourself, your nerve endings know what's coming. But when someone else touches you, the nerve endings are surprised, delighted, by a foreign hand, or whatever that hand might be holding. Besides, even if you can (and should) use a vibrator on yourself, being next to someone who is focused on your pleasure is better.

"WHAT IF YOU *NEED* THE VIBRATOR TO COME?" **A vibrator might make you orgasm faster because it is predictable, but then again, maybe it won't.**

It definitely won't turn you off the fabulous sensations of a human hand, mouth, or anything else. You will continue to like what you liked before. Variety should be your guiding principle for maximum fun. Note to women who'd never had an orgasm before they got a vibrator: the vibe may be best for you, but all orgasms start in the mind. If you can have them one way, you can have them other ways too.

1. **Even though it vibrates, you still have to move your vibrator around the clitoris, the vagina, or wherever you want it.** It may move, but it doesn't have a brain. It doesn't know what you like. (You'd be amazed how often I'm asked if moving the vibe is necessary.)

2. **Use different vibes on your partner and see what he likes. He probably won't know himself until you experiment.**

3. **If one is good, two is better. Use one on the clitoris and another in the vagina, or one in the tush during intercourse.**

4. **Reluctant vibe owners can start slowly with "intellectual alibi vibes"—the one that can double as a back or foot massager.**

5. **Make sure your partner understands you're having fun with him and what he's doing to you.** As you know, the vibrator machine isn't the point, it's who's controlling it and the fun you're having together.

6. **Consider introducing a small vibe so your partner can get used to the idea. No need to intimidate with size.** Once he understands the idea of the vibe and its limited role, it won't matter anymore what the vibe looks like.

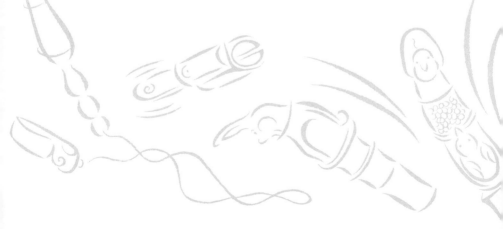

Let's Go Beyond the Buzz

Sex toys aren't just for the clitoris. Rounding out the remainder of the Safina catalog, and my personal view of what every woman should know about, consider the following items for your pleasure and delectation:

TUSH TOYS

Tush stimulators are often called "butt plugs" because of the flared base and often stubby shape. The name sounds a little harsh, but that flared base will keep the toy from slipping all the way into the tush (you don't want anything to get lost in there unless you enjoy saying, "Take me to the emergency room"). The stubby fireplug part, upon insertion in the butt, is typically designed to hit the main nerve endings in the outer inches of the rectum.

Besides plugs, the other main tush toy category is "anal beads," plastic or metal balls secured on a string, which can be inserted one at a time and then pulled out slowly at key moments (e.g., on the verge of orgasm).

DILDOS

I call the toys in this category "No Moving Parts." Not every Safina Sexory is battery operated or needs to be plugged into an outlet. Dildos are usually shaped like a penis. Many people use dildos that don't vibrate in the tush or in the vagina in conjunction with clitoral stimulation. Dildo harnesses, like underwear with a hole to put the dildo through, are made for both sexes. Women might wear a harness to stimulate their partner's prostate while doing a little role-playing. Your partner might wear the harness if you can't wait for him to recover from an orgasm. Seems like a lot of trouble to me, but whatever floats your boat rocks. Besides standard phallic-shaped dildos, we have a few curved glass or Lucite G-spot stimulators.

TIE ME UP, TIE ME DOWN

Bondage is a scary word, but issues of dominance and submission are a part of almost every relationship to some degree. Did you ever hold your lover's hands back? Well that's a hop, skip, and a jump from tying him up with a scarf. There's some excitement to be had from control and the loss of it. Some people would say that this giving and taking of control is the essence of sex. Tap into this by demystifying the would-be scary world of bondage:

Blindfolds and Cuffs. Blindfolds come in satin with faux fur lining, leather, or a synthetic material with animal prints. Lots of choice out there. Velcro or buckle cuffs are just as binding but far more comfortable than metal ones with a lock. Even without locks involved, never leave someone who is tied up alone.

Restraints. This is a serious word for scarves. Or you can get Velcro slipknot ropes that attach to the bed.

Fetish. I'm sure you've heard of people who have a shoe fetish. Most don't really, unless they need shoes to get off in bed. A fetish or paraphilia means that a person cannot experience sexual excitement without the presence of an object or activity. On a less clinical level, people throw the word around to mean they enjoy latex and rubber clothing, sensory deprivation outfits, or hoods. The most articulate spokesperson on the topic of fetish seems to be the Baroness, a fetish party host and writer in New York City. As she says of her parties, "An occasion to dress is an occasion to overdress." (For more bon mots, go to www.baroness.com.)

Sadism and masochism. Pain looms large in the thoughts of SM (as it's called by enthusiasts) players, but most say that their games are really about the power exchange between two people and the fantasy scene they're acting out. In pure SM make-believe games, there is actually little or no sex involved. First, the participants have a discussion and lay the ground rules, including the choosing of a word that, if spoken, will end the game immediately. I have interviewed dominatrixes (women who are paid to humiliate and/or hit their clients). Their clients tend to have powerful jobs. Being submissive is both a relief and thrill for them. I was told again and again that good SM, like good sex, lives in the mind. Anticipation, suspense, and uncertainty are thoughts, not deeds. SM may not be for you. I'm just throwing it out there, giving you something to think about.

More to the point, Safina carries a limited selection of SM toys for women wanting to try new things. Blindfolds with faux fur lining, patent leather cuffs that look like 1980s Madonna jewelry, and something called a "flogger" that can be used to tease or spank. We don't carry riding crops right now. Riding crops and other whips can be pretty brutal. You do need to learn what you're doing before trying advanced accessories. There's a fine line between SM and abuse. There are books on the subject and even classes throughout the SM community. As I've been saying throughout this book, the key to better sex is talking about it with other people, not reinventing the wheel. With SM this is particularly true. For more information check out *SM 101: A Realistic Introduction* by Jay Wiseman, *The New Bottoming Book* or *The New Topping Book* both by Janet W. Hardy, Dossie Easton, or the **www.sexuality.org** website. And remember to keep your tie-me-up-and-down activities about safe, consensual fun.

LOTIONS AND POTIONS
Safina offers lots of great edible massage oils, lubes, creams, chocolate body paint, and so on. They feel, smell, and taste GOOD, almost as good as the massage itself.

GAMES
There are a few fun and sexy board games out there that let you (fore)play with your partner. You'll end up sharing fantasies, making out, and having a laugh as you work your way across the board. There's even a Kama Sutra board game that will get you into the ancient positions without the tedium of reading the original three-inch thick book. A step beyond the fun of Twister all right.

BOOKS AND VIDEOS

There are hundreds of sex books out in the world. Read everything you can get your hands on. New medical discoveries are being made all the time; new possibilities constantly come out of the closet. And for every new idea or breakthrough, there'll be a book to explain it. Safina has a few literary selections available, for fun, fantasy, and function. Regarding sexy videos, Safina sells those made by women only. Porn by women is about eroticism as well as sex and is of a higher quality (lighting, attractive stars, a script that has more plot than, say, the cable guy shows up, humps three women and leaves), if still relatively low budget. You might like them the way you like a romance novel, and they might be fun to watch with your partner.

NEW THINGS AT ANY POINT IN YOUR LIFE

Sex toys for good health. There's a sales pitch you won't hear at the Dildo Hut. But it's true, and I've come a long way myself to see this truth. Using vibrators will help you to be more reliably orgasmic, thereby aiding in stress relief and flooding your body with healthful natural chemicals. More orgasms = better health. Better health = feeling energetic and happy. Feeling energetic and happy = a hotter you. A hotter you = more dates. More dates = more sex. And so on. Funny that some women may have wrongfully believed that buying a vibrator was going to hurt their motivation to date. HA!

Top Ten Ways a Vibrator Can Change Your Life

10. **You've heard that whistling while you work makes the chores seem lighter.** Consider vibrating while you work with a strap-on gizmo. You will suddenly *love* mopping. Who'd've thunk it?

9. **Takes the edge off when between boyfriends.**

8. **Takes the edge off when not between boyfriends.**

7. **They're portable. An orgasm is never farther away than a room with a lock on the door.**

6. **A vibrator orgasm gives you a morning lift. Better than coffee!**

5. **A vibrator orgasm will lull you to sleep at night. Better than Tylenol PM!**

4. **Many women have their first multiple orgasms with battery-operated help. A vibrator could lead to your breakthrough.**

3. **Vibrators never fall asleep before you come.** They don't snore either.

2. **Your partner has new ways to play with you.** And you with him.

1. **Old speed: zero to orgasm in fifteen minutes.** New speed: zero to orgasm in sixty seconds.

Five Simple Sex Toy Rules to Live By

1. **Put a condom on the sex toy for easy cleanup, but never reuse a condom or latex glove.**

2. **Do not move a sex toy from the anus to the vagina or from the vagina to the anus (use two different ones or buy two of the same one and put stickers on them to keep them separate).**

3. **Don't share a sex toy with a partner.** What's yours is yours; what's his is his.

4. **Never use silicone-based lube on a silicone sex toy because it will degrade the toy.**

5. **Sex toys are like clothes.** Choose your toy depending on your mood, what fits well that day, and what feels comfortable.

Sex Toy Care and Maintenance

* **Use warm water and mild soap.** Don't get the batteries wet. Pat or air dry.

* **If it is waterproof, you can get the whole thing wet.**

* **Silicone or glass products that don't have moving parts can be put in the dishwasher.**

* **Baby wipes often contain chemicals that degrade sex toy material.** Don't use them.

* **Condoms make for easy cleanup.** Condoms really stretch and can be put over odd-shaped toys too.

Afterglow

It doesn't matter how old or experienced you are, what religion, orientation, ethnicity, financial status, marital status. Whoever you are, talking openly and honestly about your sex life will improve it. The more you talk, the more you learn. The more you learn, the more confident and comfortable you will become with both the topic of discussion and the act itself (or I should say, "acts themselves"). You'd be surprised how even the smallest piece of information can make a big difference. Even knowing that other women have had similar sexual experiences—good and bad— will be a comfort. *You are not alone!* You've never been alone with your concerns and questions about sex. Everything I do now—with my company and this book—is to show women that sharing sexual experiences and information among friends will enrich all of our sex lives (and overall health, if I haven't fully exhausted that point yet).

The stories below help illustrate my point. Each is true, a confession made to me or to a Safina Specialist at a Salon (with one exception). I call this chapter "Afterglow," because that's how I feel after giving a Safina Salon presentation, and apparently, so do the women who attended, telling me, as they pack up their bags, "Wow. That was great for me. Was it good for you too?" My answer is always an unequivocal, "Yes! Yes! *YES!!!!!!*"

"I've never told anyone this before, but . . ."

Sarah is a 32-year-old writer who's had the same boyfriend for five years. She attended a Safina Salon in New York City. When I got to the G-spot part, she said, "So it can feel like you're going to pee when someone finds it?" You should have seen her expression. It was like a lightbulb went off over her head. She said, "If only I knew then what I know now."

I asked her to elaborate. She said, "I've never told anyone about this before. It was a year ago. My boyfriend and I were having a great night. We were having the best sex of our lives. I don't know if it was the mood or the foreplay. But it all came together that night. I was lying on my stomach, and he was behind me. It was a strange angle. Different for us. After a while, I felt a big orgasm starting to build. The feeling was overwhelming, like I didn't know what was happening to me. Just as I was about to come, I felt like I had to pee. I seized up and lost the feeling completely. It was there, I panicked about peeing, and then it was gone. I've been chasing that feeling every time we've had sex for another year, but the fear of peeing always keeps me from getting there."

She never told anyone about this experience because she was embarrassed. She thought she was going to be incontinent in bed when what was really happening was the building up of a powerful G-spot orgasm. Now that she's learned about the G-spot, its connection to the urethral sponge, and its "about to pee" sensation, Sarah couldn't stop smiling. And she was one of the first women to leave the Salon that night. I'm quite certain where she was rushing off to.

"Sex is something you do, not something you talk about."

Shortly after I got Safina off the ground, I met Jane, a successful businesswoman in her 60s, at a conference. At a lunch with several other women, Jane looked extremely disapproving when I explained the mission of Safina. The other women at the table asked me a litany of enthusiastic questions. Jane kept her eyes down and ate her salad quietly. Later, on the way out of the restaurant, I asked if she was offended by the discussion about sex. She said indignantly, "I wasn't offended. I just don't know what all the fuss is about. Sex is something you do, not something you talk about." I knew then that she'd been raised in the old tradition of shame and silence about sex as most women of her generation were. The conference continued, but I couldn't shake what I could have said to Jane to put her more at ease. The subject of sex is simply too huge to relegate to the category of "not something you talk about."

I ran into Jane later that day in the hotel lobby. She must have been thinking about our lunch too. She said, "I wasn't raised in this culture of openness. I grew up in a very strict Catholic family, and we didn't talk about anything."

"The last thing I meant to do was make you uncomfortable," I said.

"You didn't. I just didn't know how to participate in the conversation." She paused (I've come to notice that there is always a pause before a woman makes a big confession) and said, "I can't believe I'm going to tell you this, but I have a problem right now, and I don't know what to do or whom to talk to."

Conversations like this make me love my job. I said, "You can talk to me." I shut up and listened, having figured out that listening is often the best way to help.

"I have fallen in love with a man who is much older than me—and I'm not so young myself," she said. "He's the most interesting, fantastic person I've ever met, and he feels the same way about me." She was suddenly glowing and her previously pursed lips were now framing a huge, enthusiastic grin.

Her smile was contagious, and I beamed back at her. "That's wonderful! Congratulations!" I said.

"Well, there's one problem." She looked around to see if anyone was within earshot before leaning in and saying, "He doesn't know how to satisfy me in bed. He's old and quite delicate. Maybe you can suggest something for us to take the pressure off of him. I may seem uptight and conservative, but I do think about sex a lot, and I'm not willing to live the rest of my life without it. I love him but I can't stay in this relationship unless I can still have sex."

I didn't know what to say for a minute. I wanted her late-in-life love to succeed, and I agreed with her that sex was an important factor in any relationship's success. She added, "We're going away this weekend, and if we can't make sex work somehow, I'm going to have to break up with him. Do you have anything I can try?"

I said, "I've got a lot of things for you. Why don't we look at them together? But I am concerned about his fragility. You need to speak to his doctor before you use anything on him."

"I've been asking his doctor questions about this," Jane said. "I'll call him and check on anything before we go away. I really want to make this work. I want him to be able to make me happy in bed. He feels as bad about it as I do."

We went to my room. I spread out my vibrator samples on the bed and showed her my catalog. We talked about different lubricants, the clitoris, the G-spot, and how to bring Sexories into a relationship without being intimidating. I put batteries in everything, and we talked about the different designs.

"I can't believe I'm shopping for sex toys," said Jane at one point. "I just can't believe this." She picked two vibrators and some lubricant. I delivered them to her personally the next day (I didn't have a ware-house with shipping capacity back then).

On Monday, the first day back from their weekend, Jane called me. "You saved our relationship!" she said as soon as I picked up the phone. She went on to tell me that her beau was thrilled she brought something fun along on the trip. As we'd discussed that day, she'd presented the Sexories as exciting surprises, and that's just how they were received. They laughed, played, had a great, repeatedly satisfying time with them. They were both thrilled, she said. "I was going to call you anyway to let you know what happened, but you know, he asked me if I'd call and thank you for him."

Nothing could be more gratifying. Making sex information and products accessible does change people's lives. If I had any doubts about Safina, they were squashed. I'd found my calling.

"I have a WHAT???"

Kim read about Safina Salons in her local paper, *The Salt Lake City Tribune*. She looked me up on the Internet and said she wanted to join the Safina team. Kim is happily married and passionately agrees with Safina's mission—to make sex a normal topic of conversation. Kim lives in a part of the country that is particularly silent about sex and yet values happy marriage as a central goal. As far as she can see, the lack of sex information and discussion is antithetical to having a happy marriage.

Kim's Salon-goers are frequently religious Mormons. The majority of these women got married in their early 20s and have received little or no sex education. Kim, a mid-30s mother of two, grew up a Mormon as well, so she knew exactly what she would be dealing with.

Lisa, a 38-year-old mother of two, is a typical attendee at Kim's Salons. She'd been married for sixteen years when she came to a Salon with her mother and sister-in-law. Kim was taking them through some of the information covered in this book, smiling and laughing as she told her own stories.

"The whole group was hanging onto my every word," Kim told me at the time. "They didn't eat, they didn't drink. They were spellbound. I could see that things were flashing through their minds as I talked about the clitoris, where it is, how it's structured like a penis but has more nerve endings. Lisa and the other women were concentrating hard on what I was saying. Clearly, they hadn't heard anything about this before.

"I'm used to the intense silence, which is so different from the Safina Salons I have been to outside of this area," continued Kim. "The Utah women need to be encouraged to ask questions. They don't shout them out spontaneously. So when I finished talking about the clitoris, I asked them if they have any questions. Lisa, who'd been stunned motionless and silent for my whole talk, jumped out of her chair and started shouting, 'How is it that no one ever told me that I had a clitoris? I'm 38 years old with two kids, and I have no idea what's going on down there. Did anyone else here know this stuff? How could I be this old and not know anything?'"

Those were bigger questions than, "How many nerve endings did you say?" Kim never got a chance to attempt to answer Lisa, since her outburst immediately set everyone else off. The women present started sharing their stories, telling each other about their confusion and what little they had figured out up until now.

"We were strangers when we met, but when we said goodbye at the end of the Salon, we hugged and some women teared up with emotion," said Kim. "I hope that they are each having a great time getting to know the parts of themselves they literally didn't know existed. I know they all have Safina Sexories now to explore with. And I hope that the next sixteen years of Lisa's marital bliss includes lots of clitoral bliss too."

"I didn't know that wasn't normal."

Usually, Safina Salons are fun and cheerful. But every now and then, upon hearing friends talk about their husbands and boyfriends, a woman realizes that she hasn't been treated well by her partner. Jeanine, 25, was such a woman.

We were on the subject of tush sex. Jeanine listened to her friends talking about their experiences, and she couldn't believe what she was hearing. "How can any of you say you like it?" she asked. "Anal sex hurts! It's horrible. Every time my boyfriend does it, I'm in pain for a week."

The room went silent for a second. Jeanine's friend Carrie asked, "What does he do exactly?"

Jeanine recounted how her boyfriend gets excited and shoves his penis into her butt. No lubricant, no foreplay, and no discussion with her along the way. "He doesn't go slow, wait for the tush to open up. None of the stuff you're talking about here, and I don't think there's any way he ever would. I can't believe that any man would. He likes it the way he does it."

Jeanine's friends sent e-mails after the Salon thanking me for opening up that discussion. In post-Salon conversations with Jeanine, they all came to realize that she was in an abusive relationship. Jeanine told them that she always thought everyone was dealing with those same issues in relationships that she was. It never crossed her mind to talk to her friends about her extremely rough and insensitive boyfriend because she just assumed that he was normal and she wasn't. This group of women had been friends for more than ten years, but they never knew what Jeanine was going through. Women often decide that when they feel they aren't being treated right that they somehow brought it on themselves or deserve it. Women provide each other with important support. Friends will take care of you, especially when a partner does not. Jeanine's Salon lesson may have changed her attitude about sex. It may have changed the course of her life.

"I've never had an orgasm."

Sylvia is a successful attorney in a large firm by day. By evening, she is a Safina Specialist. She believes strongly in the mission of the company, plus she enjoys conducting Salons. The extra income doesn't hurt. Sylvia has an expensive shoe habit. Selling sex toys on the side keeps her in Jimmy Choos.

At one of her first Salons, Sylvia met Leslie, a 34-year-old woman who confessed that she'd never had an orgasm. She'd been married for ten years, had a 5-year-old son, and was starting to give up hope that she'd ever figure out what all this orgasm fuss was about. She said, "My husband and I have tried every position, every possible oral and manual means. I've tried masturbating too. After a while, it starts to hurt, and then there's no chance in hell it's going to happen. Sex has become a big letdown. Not just for me, but my husband is also frustrated. I'm on the verge of accepting that I'm never going to have one." The Salon attendees gave her the good advice to relax and not see orgasm as a goal. Sylvia recommended her favorite combination of Sexories—the Crystal Wand (a curved piece of Lucite designed to hit the G-spot) plus a Blueberry I-Vibe for the clitoris.

Leslie and her husband called Sylvia a week later and left a joint voicemail yelling "THANK YOU" into Sylvia's answering machine. Leslie had her first orgasm with her new sex toys. She'd had several, actually, and told Sylvia she plans to make up for lost time.

Sylvia replayed the message again and again. She felt like dancing in her Jimmy Choos. "No matter how great Leslie's orgasm was, it probably wasn't better than how I felt for being able to help her," she told me.

"Don't hate. Masturbate."

Shameka is another Safina Specialist, dedicated to improving the sex life of every woman she meets. She hosted her first Salon, inviting twenty friends and colleagues, ranging in age from 25 to 35. Shameka asked everyone to talk a little bit about themselves first. A third had kids and all but two were married or had boyfriends. The whole group participated in the discussion from beginning to end, and Shameka was amazed at how much she learned about the women she thought she knew so well.

One woman, Garnetta, had gotten a divorce six years ago and was raising two little kids on her own. Shameka and their mutual friends at the Salon knew that she didn't have a boyfriend but they assumed she was dating now and then but that she hadn't met anyone special enough to mention. Garnetta asked if a vibrator would turn her off to men when she finally got another one.

Everyone jumped in with comments on this, "What are you saying, Garnetta? You're afraid you'll get hooked on a machine that doesn't talk back, doesn't forget to call you, and doesn't do anything but exactly what you want it to?" And, "I love my vibrators but I love my man too. Find a man with an open mind, and you don't have to choose."

Garnetta stopped the crowd from going on, "No, no you don't understand. I haven't had sex in a *very* long time."

"How long?" everyone shouted at once.

"Six years," Garnetta answered.

There was a hush. Everyone was a little shocked. "Damn," someone said.

"Don't feel bad for me," Garnetta said. "No, no, no. I'm fine. I have a saying, for whenever I think about my ex, and how I haven't met someone else. I say, 'Don't hate, masturbate.' And you know I feel great. I'd like to meet a good man, but until then I know how to take care of me."

Twenty women started laughing and chanting Garnetta's saying. Shameka told her, "I'm so proud of you. Thinking so positively, and going through what you're going through." All the women agreed and assured Garnetta that she'd be fine when the right guy came along. Someone suggested the group get t-shirts with her saying on them. It was declared the theme of the night, and a toast to Garnetta was proposed. "To Garnetta our hero—no, our heroine! Think positive! Don't Hate, Masturbate!"

"Here comes the bride."

Bridal showers are a good excuse for a Safina Salon. They are always fun, and often touching. Kelly's best friend Melissa was getting married in a month, and so she had all their childhood and college friends over for an elegant summer barbecue. She made roasted corn salad, grilled salmon, and cookies. The guests were asked to send pictures of the bride in advance. Kelly made a slideshow on her laptop, and she started the Salon with this pictorial review of Melissa's life. She's an extremely successful accountant at a large firm and has worked tirelessly at her job while keeping all these wonderful friends. They talked about what it was like when Melissa met John years ago in college and how much they approved of her choice of him.

Then Kelly had each one of their friends go around and tell Melissa their wish for her marriage. Everyone was crying and laughing and smiling at once. One friend said she wished that Melissa would be able to get John out of the habit of putting his muddy mountain bike in the closet with her suits. Another said she wished Melissa would find a way to live with his beer fridge (apparently, the appliance was covered in stickers he'd been collecting since age 18). Another hoped Melissa would always be as happy with John as she had been for the last six years. Their wishes were simple and moving.

When it was Kelly's turn, she said, "Melissa, what I wish for you, my best friend since second grade, is that you will continue to live your life with all your heart and your fearless passion. You moved across the country to go to school and fell in love with John. You've gone through a huge move for your job and John was right there for you with every new adventure. I know you'll continue to discover new things about each other. More than anything, I'm sure that you keep expanding on your fabulous sex life, that the phrase 'here comes the bride' will apply to you for every day of your married life. That's why I had a Safina Salon for your bridal shower. I hope you'll enjoy each other in every way you can every single day for the rest of your lives. That is my wish for you."

What I wish for you

What I wish for you: keep learning, exploring, and talking about sex. Too many people can tell a stylist exactly how to cut their hair but can't tell the partner who loves them what to do in bed. Communication is the only trick in this sex book—or any sex book. Great sex and deep intimacy, you can have it all. But first, try saying three little words: "I was thinking . . ."

So. This is the end. I've said enough. It's time to close the book. Admire my photo on the back cover for a moment. Make a note of my e-mail address to send me your thoughts. And then, go put all you've learned into practice.

I wish you the best sex you'll ever have. Each and every day. Each and every way.

Sources and Resources

ABOUT THE CLITORIS

Angier, Natalie. 1996. Ideas and trends: Intersexual healing: An anomaly finds a group. *New York Times*, February 4, Week in Review, p.14.

Bartholinus, Thomas. 1651. *Anatomia ex Caspari Bartholini parentis institionibus*. Paris: Bibliothèque nationale.

Bellinger, Mark F. 1993. Subtotal de-epithelialization and partial concealment of the glans clitoris: A modification to improve the cosmetic results of feminizing genitoplasty. *Journal of Urology* 150: 651–53.

Bonaparte, Marie. 1953. *Female Sexuality*. Grove Press, New York, NY.

Caprio, Frank S. 1953. *The Sexually Adequate Female*. Fawcett Gold Medal Books, Greenwich, CT. Reprint 1966.

Chalker, Rebecca. 2000. *Clitoral Truth: The World at Your Fingertips*. Seven Stories Press, New York, NY.

Clitoris Web site: http://the-clitoris.com.

Coleman, Sarah. 2002. Female parts. *World Press Review*, June 6.

Dally, Ann. 1991. *Women under the Knife: A History of Surgery*. London: Hutchinson Radius.

Edgerton, Milton T. 1993. Discussion: Clitoroplasty for clitoromegaly due to adrenogenital syndrome without loss of sensitivity. *Plastic and Reconstructive Surgery* 91: 956.

Ellis, Albert. 1958. *Sex without Guilt*. Grove Press, New York, NY. Reprint 1965.

Online Etymology Dictionary (for the history of the word "clitoris"): http://www.Etymonline.com.

Feibleman, Peter. 1997. Natural causes. *DoubleTake Magazine*. Winter. http://www.fictionwriter.com/double.htm.

Gearhart, John P., Arthur Burnett, and Jeffrey Owen. 1995. Measurement of evoked potentials during feminizing genitoplasty: technique and applications. *Journal of Urology* 153: 486–87.

Gross, Robert E., Judson Randolph, and John F. Crigler. 1966. Clitorectomy for sexual abnormalities: Indications and technique. *Surgery* 59: 300–308.

Kinsey, Alfred C. 1953. *Sexual Behavior in the Human Female*. Pocket Books, New York, NY. 1973 reprint.

Kobelt, G.L. 1884. Die Männlichen und Weiblichen. *Wollusts-Organe des Menschen und verschiedene Saugetiere*. Paris: Bibliothèque nationale.

Koedt, Anne. 1970. *The Myth of the Vaginal Orgasm*. Reprinted in full on the Chicago Women's Liberation Union Herstory Web site. http://www.cwluherstory.com/CWLUArchive/classic.html.

Litwin, A., I. Aitkin, and P. Merlob. 1990. Clitoral length assessment in newborn infants of 30 to 41 weeks gestational age. *European Journal of Obstetrics and Gynecology and Reproductive Biology* 38: 209–12.

Masters and Johnson. 1966. *Human Sexual Response*. Little, Brown, Boston, MA.

Oberfield, Sharon E., Aurora Mondok, Farrokh Shahrivar, Janice F. Klein, and Lenore S. Levine. 1989. Clitoral size in full-term infants. *American Journal of Perinatology* 6: 453–54.

O'Connell, Helen E. 1998. Anatomical relationship between urethra and clitoris. *Journal of Urology* 159: 1892. Synopsis of original article at http://www.infotrieve.com/freemedline/.

Randolph, Judson, and Wellington Hung. 1970. Reduction clitoroplasty in females with hypertrophied clitoris. *Journal of Pediatric Surgery* 5: 224–30.

University of Melbourne, Department of Anatomy and Cell Biology. http://www.anatomy.unimelb.edu.au/.

Williamson, Susan. 1998. The Truth about Women. *New Scientist*. http://www.newscientist.com/ns/980801/women.html.

ORGANIZATIONS FOR INFORMATION AND ACTIVISM

Female Genital Cutting Education and Networking Project: http://www.fgmnetwork.org/index.php.

Intersex Society of North America (ISNA) is a great resource for information about clitoral "reductions" on infants and children in the United States: http://www.isna.org/.

National Organization for Women: http://www.now.org.

V-DAY (and *The Vagina Monologues*): http://www.vday.org/main.html.

World Health Organization: http://www.who.int/health_topics/ female_genital_mutilation/en/.

THE G-SPOT

Gräfenberg, Ernest. 1950. The Role of the Urethra in Female Orgasm. *International Journal of Sexology*. 3:3 145–148.

Jones, Nicola. 2002. Bigger is better when it comes to the G spot. *New Scientist*, July 3. http://www.newscientist.com/news/news.jsp?id=ns99992495.

Perry, John D. The Paraurethral, or "Skene's Glands" in Scientific Literature. Selected views. http://www.incontinet.com/skenesgland.htm.

Whipple, Beverly, John D. Perry, and Alice Kahn Ladas. 1983. *The G Spot and Other Discoveries about Human Sexuality*. Revised edition. Dell, New York, NY.

Zaviacic, Milan, M.D. 1999. *The Human Female Prostate*. Bratislava: Slovak Academic Press.

Zaviacic M., Ablin R.J. 2000. The female prostate and prostate-specific antigen. Immunohistochemical localization, implications of this prostate marker in women and reasons for using the term "prostate" in the human female. *Histol Histopathol* 15: 131–42.

FEMALE ORGASMS

Angier, Natalie. 2000. *Women: An Intimate Geography*. Anchor Books, New York, NY.

Blakemore, Colin, and Sheila Jennett. 2001. *The Oxford Companion to the Body*. Oxford: Oxford University Press.

Bodansky, Steve, and Vera Bodansky. 2002. *Illustrated Guide to Extended Massive Orgasm.* Hunter House, CA.

Carroll, E. Jean. 1984. Frigid women. *Playboy*, April 1984.

Cattrall, Kim, Mark Levinson, and Fritz Drury. 2003. *Satisfaction: The Art of the Female Orgasm.* Warner Books, New York, NY.

Clarkson, Petruska. 2002. False Facts(?). *IPNOSIS*, November 7, 2002. http://ipnosis.postle.net/pages/PClarksonFalseFacts.htm.

Dodson, Betty. 1974. *Liberating Masturbation.* Self-published.

———. 1996. *Sex for One: The Joy of Self-Loving.* Three Rivers Press, New York, NY.

Foucault, Michel. 1980. *The History of Sexuality.* Vintage Books, New York, NY.

Freud, Sigmund. 1910. The origin and development of psychoanalysis. *American Journal of Psychology* 21: 181–218.

———. 1914. *The History of the Psychoanalytic Movement.* Translation by A. A. Brill. First published in 1917 in the *Nervous and Mental Disease Monograph Series 25*. Nervous and Mental Disease Publishing, New York.

———. 1933. Lecture XXXV (1932): A philosophy of life. *New Introductory Lectures on Psycho-analysis.* Hogarth Press, London.

Kline-Graber, Georgia, and Benjamin Graber. 1975. *A Guide to Sexual Satisfaction: Women's Orgasm.* Warner Books, New York, NY.

Kolata, Gina. 1998. Women and sex: On this topic, science blushes. *New York Times*, June 21. http://www.nytimes.com/partners/aol/special/women/nyt98/.

Lydon, Susan. 1968. Understanding orgasm. *Ramparts Magazine.* Reprint by Hip Publishing January 15, 2002. http://www.hippy.com/article.php?sid=92.

Maines, Rachel P. 1999. *The Technology of Orgasm: "Hysteria," the Vibrator, and Women's Sexual Satisfaction.* Baltimore: Johns Hopkins University Press.

Morantz-Sanchez, Regina. 2000. *Sympathy and Science: Women Physicians in American Medicine.* Chapel Hill: University of North Carolina Press.

Paget, Lou. 2000. *How to Give Her Absolute Pleasure: Totally Explicit Techniques Every Woman Wants Her Man to Know.* Broadway Books, New York, NY.

PENIS AND PROSTATE

Bechtel, Stefan. 1998. *Sex: A Man's Guide.* Men's Health. Rodale Press, Emmaus, PA.

Chia, Mantak, Todd Buck, and Douglas Abrams Arava. 1997. *The Multi-Orgasmic Man: Sexual Secrets Every Man Should Know.* Illus. Todd Buck. HarperSanFrancisco, San Francisco, CA.

da Ros, C., et al. 1994. Caucasian penis: What is the Normal Size? *Journal of Urology* 151: 323A [abstract 381].

Gilbaugh, James H. 1989. *A Doctor's Guide to Men's Private Parts.* Crown Publishers, New York, NY.

Gonzales, Gustavo F. 2001. Function of seminal vesicles and their role in male fertility. *Asian Journal of Andrology* 3: 251–58.

Kinsey Institute. 1990. *The Kinsey Institute New Report on Sex.* St. Martin's Press, New York, NY.

Masters, W.H., and V.E. Johnson. 1966. *Human Sexual Response.* Little, Brown, Boston, MA.

Phillip, M., et al. 1996. Clitoral and penile sizes of full term newborns in two different ethnic groups. *Journal of Pediatric Endocrinology and Metabolism* 9: 175–9.

THE TUSH

Morin, Jack. 2000. *Anal Pleasure and Health: A Guide for Men and Women.* Revised edition. Down There Press, San Francisco, CA.

Taormino, Tristan. 1997. *The Ultimate Guide to Anal Sex for Women.* Cleis Press, San Francisco, CA.

GENERAL SEX AND TECHNIQUE

Anderson, Dan, and Maggie Berman. 1997. *Sex Tips for Straight Women from a Gay Man*. Regan Books, New York, NY.

Blume, Judy. 1976. *Forever . . .* Simon & Schuster, New York, NY.

———. 1971. *Are You There God? It's Me, Margaret*. Bantam Doubleday Dell Books for Young Readers, New York, NY. 1971 reissue.

Boteach, Schumley. 2000. *Kosher Sex: A Recipe for Passion and Intimacy*. Main Street Books, New York, NY.

Chang, Jolan, and Jolan Chung. 1977. *Tao of Love and Sex: The Ancient Chinese Way to Ecstasy*. Penguin, New York, NY.

Dickinson, Robert Latou. 1949. *Atlas of Human Sex Anatomy*. Baltimore: Williams and Wilkins.

Diamond, Jared. 1998. *Why Is Sex Fun?: The Evolution of Human Sexuality*. Basic Books, New York, NY.

Joannides, Paul. 2000. *The Guide to Getting It On! (The Universe's Coolest and Most Informative Book about Sex)*. Goofy Foot Press, Worldport, OR.

Keesling, Barbara. 2001. *The Good Girl's Guide to Bad Girl Sex*. M. Evans & Co., New York, NY.

Lacroix, Nitya, and Mark Harwood. 1997. *The Art of Tantric Sex*. DK Publishing, New York, NY.

Michael, Robert T., Edward O. Laumann, John H. Gagnon, and Gina Bari Kolata. 1995. *Sex in America: A Definitive Survey*. Warner Books, New York, NY.

Netter, Frank H., and John T. Hansen. 2002. *Atlas of Human Anatomy*. Icon Learning Systems, Teterboro, NY.

Paget, Lou. 2001. *The Big O*. Broadway Books, New York, NY.

Reuben, David. 2000. *Everything You Always Wanted to Know about Sex (But Were Afraid to Ask)*. St. Martin's Press, New York, NY.

The World's Best Anatomical Charts. 2000. Anatomical Chart Company, Skokie, IL.

Wiseman, Jay. 1996. *SM 101: A Realistic Introduction*. Greenery Press, San Francisco, CA.

Acknowledgments

Shannon Mullen would like to thank her mother, Sheila Finch, for all her support; all the Safina Specialists; and the many Salon attendees who've contributed to this book and to Safina's growth. Thank you to all the people who shared their experiences and expertise on sex, health, and relationships. And thank you Val Frankel, Julie Merberg, and Kristin Kiser at Crown.

Val Frankel would like to thank Shannon Mullen, Julie Merberg, and Kristin Kiser.

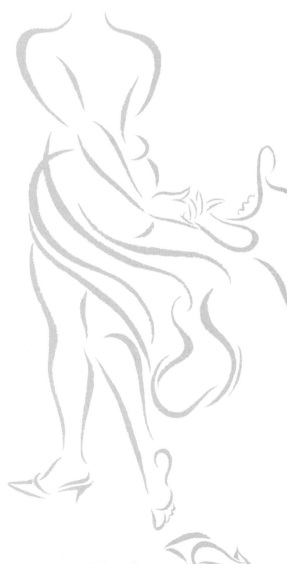